# HEALTHY SEEDS FOR SWEET FRUITS

## VIJAY KULKARNI

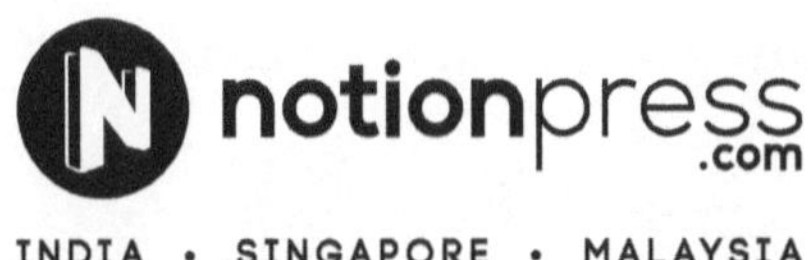

INDIA · SINGAPORE · MALAYSIA

# Notion Press

No. 8, 3rd Cross Street
CIT Colony, Mylapore
Chennai, Tamil Nadu – 600004

First Published by Notion Press 2020
Copyright © Vijay Kulkarni 2020
All Rights Reserved.

ISBN 978-1-64983-830-8

# Contents

# Prologue

---

I am pleased to present my fourth book in series of 'Medical Astrology" to all my beloved readers and friends. With respect to the first book in this series "Horoscope of Stethoscope" I have no words to express my feelings and emotions for the overwhelming response you had given to my book. And the same response for my second Book "Uterus Scanned Under Horoscope" Particularly my Doctor friends working world over for Humanity had extended the unexpected extra support and guidance for further work which I am sure I neither can put in words nor can I express my deep gratitude for their hearty response. My third title "Fate of the Fetus" also received great response from my doctor friends, and this time another title "Healthy Seeds for Sweat Fruits" I am sure you shall like.

There is a proverb said, "If soil and seeds are perfect the fruits certainly come with extra sweet"and as such some cases of female ill health are well discussed in this book.

In this presentation again I am trying to contain some more elaborative connections between planetary disposition thereby trying to understand the exact cause and orientation of the disease related to Uterus and unborn child. In our society it is observed often that any disease or disorder related to Uterus is ignored till it becomes cause of infertility and or it becomes major cause of physical ailment that is likely to be a threat to life. In this work of collection of medical information, case studies and growth of disease over passage of time was difficult and was only possible due to unlimited and uncensored cooperation from my medical fraternity. Therefore, it becomes very much necessary to express my heartiest thanks and feelings for all the doctors specifically those who have worked with me to assess every case with respect to the horoscope, Birth chart and current planetary status. With investment of small time on study of birth chart can yield bright results and major life threats or birth of spastic child or Child with Autism can be avoided.

Also, I am very much excited to express my sincere and cordial thanks to all my clients who had approached me and offered very cooperation in this regard. I also cannot forget to express my sincere thanks and obligations to those whom I have not seen but they have helped me a lot in this venture including Encyclopaedias Britannica and others.

**Vijay Kulkarni**
(Author)

# Epigraph

I wondered how I can make her speak who remained in front of me invisible and drives me to work persistently!

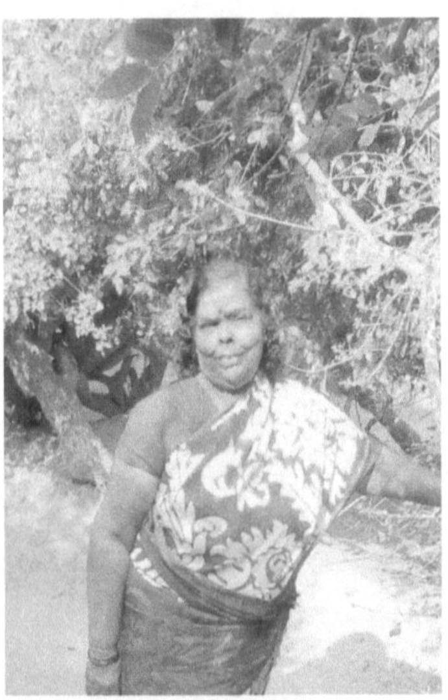

SAU. VIDYA VIJAY KULKARNI

# Chapter 1

# Gamut of Female Health

The link we have studied in our schooldays that unlike other mammals, human reproductive system is most evolved and advanced; and as such we all the human are most cautious and concerned about our health but unfortunately most often female health is given secondary importance rather ignored totally. This happens not only in illiterate and unprivileged society but is observed in even highly civilized and learned society. Female experiences micro aggression as gender bias behaviour by male in the society. Also, gender disparities in medical health care are recorded. Though the normal low belly pains are common and normal during pregnancy; however, many women even in their adolescence ages experience pain in lower belly which is ignored assuming it is common in all females. UTIs are relatively common in females, like burning sensation while urinating, feeling extremely tired, shaky with cranky mood are few signs when females are required to seek medical attention but due to the social reasons and also sort of inferiority complex about being female these complaints are totally negated or ignored. Also, it is assumed unethical to discuss about uterine health with parents and this causes further aggravation of the disorders.

Most often we observe women ignore dysfunctional bleeding or pelvic pains because they think it is normal but in reality these symptoms can be signs of abnormal cell growth or fibroid growth, polyps growth, or infection or even structured and functional disorders that occur even in adolescent age group uterus is also known as the womb, a major female reproductive organ of female body.

The uterus is located within pelvic region immediately behind and almost overlying the bladder and in front of sigmoid colon. The uterus is developed from para meso nephric duct. The human uterus is pear shaped and about 7.6-centimeter-long and 4.5 centimeter broad and about 3.0 thick. Atypical uterus weighs about 60 grams. The uterus can automatically be divided into four regions. The Fundus, or uppermost rounded portion of the uterus; the corpus (body), the cervix and the cervical canal.

The cervix protrudes into the vaginal vault; the uterus is hold in position within the pelvis by ligaments which are part of endo- pelvic foscia. These ligaments include the pubo cervical ligament, the cardinal ligaments and the utero sacral ligaments. It is covered by sheet like fold of peritoneum, the broad ligaments.

From outside to inside the region of ligaments includes

1.   Cervix of uterus
2.   External orifice of uterus
3.   Cervical canal
4.   Internal orifice of uterus
5.   Body or corpus uterus
6.   Uterine cavity
7.   Fundus

**Layers**

The uterus has three layers which together form uterine wall. From innermost to outermost these layers are endometrial layer, Myometrium and Perimetrium; the endometrial layer is the inner epithelial layer along with its mucous membrane. It has basal layers and the functional layers; the functional layer thickens and then is sloughed off during menstrual cycle or estrous cycle. During pregnancy, the uterine glands and blood vessels in the endometrial layer further increase in size and numbers to form the deciduous vascular spaces fuse and become interconnected to form placenta which supplies oxygen and nutritious fluid to embryo in fetus. The myometrial layer uterus mostly consists of smooth muscles. The innermost layer of myometrium is known as the junction zone which becomes thickened in Adenomyosis.

The peritoneum is serous layer of visceral covers outer surface of the uterus. Surrounding the uterus is layer of band of fibrous and fatty connective tissue called perimetrium that connects the uterus to other tissues of pelvis. Commensal organisms are present in the uterus and form uterine micro biome.

The uterus is primarily supported by pelvic diaphragm, perineal body and urogenital diaphragm. Secondarily it is supported by ligaments including the peritoneal ligament and the broad ligament of uterus.

## Cervix

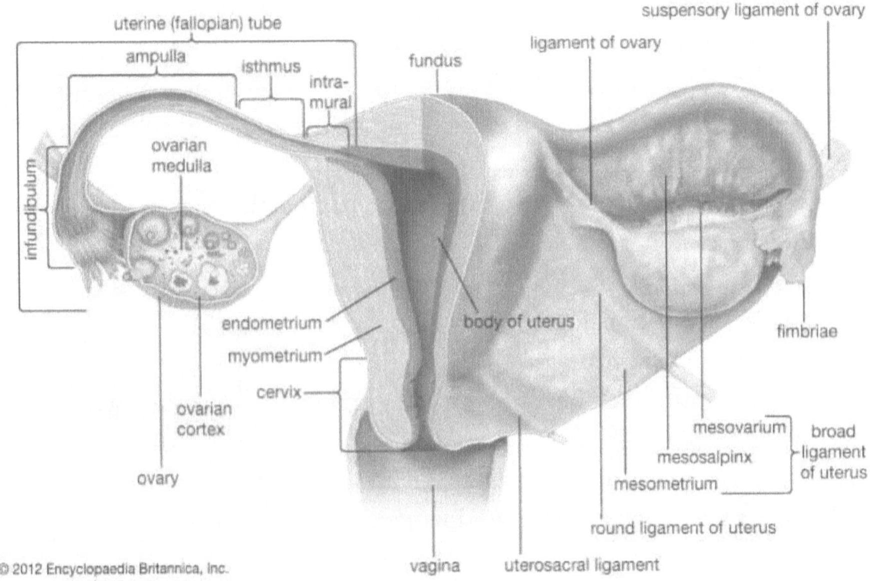


Normally uterus lies in ante version and ante flexion; in most cases the long axis of the uterus is bent forward on the long axis of vagina against the urinary bladder; this position is referred as Ante version of uterus. Furthermore, the long axis is bent forward at the level of the internal os with the long axis of cervix. The uterus assumes ante verted position in 50% of women; retroverted position in 25% women and midposed position in remaining 25% women. The uterus is in middle of the pelvic cavity and is mobile and moves posteriorly under pressure of full bladder; anteriorly under pressure of full rectum and if both are full it moves upwards.

Increased intra-abdominal pressure pushes it down wards and this mobility is conferred to uterus by musculo fibrous apparatus that consists of suspensor and sustentacular part. Under normal circumstances the suspensory part keeps the uterus in ante version in 90% women and keeps floating in the pelvic region.

The blood supply to uterus is supplied by uterine artery and ovarian artery, and uterine vein and ovarian vein. The nerve supply i.e. sympathetic nerve supply is from hypo gastric plexus and the ovarian plexus. Parasympathetic nerve supply is from S2, S3, and S4 nerves.

Bilateral Mullerian ducts form during early period of fetal life. In males Antimulerian hormone is secreted from testis that leads to their regression. In females these ducts give rise to the fallopian tubes, Ovaries and the uterus. In case of uterine malfunction this development may be disturbed. The body's autonomic nervous system which regulates "automated" metabolic processes such as heart rate, breathing, digestion and sexual arousal also has links with the uterus, breasts and brain.

Clinical significance of the uterus; some pathological states

1. Prolapsed of uterus
2. Carcinoma of cervix, malignant neoplasm.
3. Carcinoma malignant neoplasm
4. Fibroids, benign neoplasm.
5. Adenomyosis, ectopic growth of endometrial tissue within the myometrium.
6. Pyometra, infection of uterus at the uterine cavity.
7. Endometritis, infection in uterine cavity.
8. Uterine malformation mainly congenital.
9. Rokitansky syndrome (congenital absence of uterus)
10. Aschermann's syndrome. I.e. intra uterine adhesions.
11. Hematometra i.e. accumulation of blood within uterus.
12. Mesometritis inflame of muscular uterine wall.

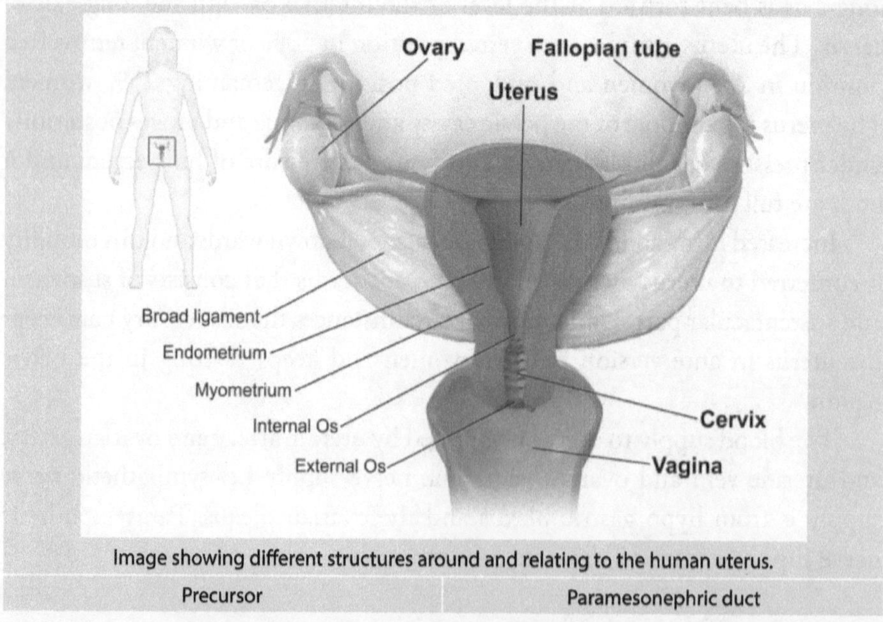


Image showing different structures around and relating to the human uterus.

| Precursor | Paramesonephric duct |
| --- | --- |

Normally, the uterus lies in anteversion and anteflexion. In most women, the long axis of the uterus is bent forward on the long axis of the vagina, against the urinary bladder. This position is referred to as anteversion of the uterus. Furthermore, the long axis of the body of the uterus is bent forward at the level of the internal os with the long axis of the cervix. This position is termed anteflexion of the uterus. The uterus assumes an anteverted position in 50% of women, a retroverted position in 25% of women, and a midposed position in the remaining 25% of women.

## Position

The uterus is in the middle of the pelvic cavity in frontal plane (due to ligamentum latum uteri). The fundus does not surpass the linea terminalis, while the vaginal part of the cervix does not extend below the interspinal line. The uterus is mobile and moves posteriorly under the pressure of a full bladder, or anteriorly under the pressure of a full rectum. If both are full, it moves upwards. Increased intra-abdominal pressure pushes it downwards. The mobility is conferred to it by Musculo-fibrous apparatus that consists of suspensory and sustentacular part. Under normal circumstances the suspensory part keeps the uterus in anteflexion and anteversion (in 90% of women) and keeps it "floating" in the pelvis.

# Chapter 2

# Lords of Cusp for Uterus

If we draw a birth chart of any femalenative, we can find out that fifth cusp in the birth chart from ascendant gives detailed information regarding intelligence, planning skills, cognitive abilities and detailed functioning or malfunctioning of uterus. It is referred to as house of happiness on account of children; and as such we have considered only this aspect of fifth cusp in our all discussions in this book. While considering we may have to assess and understand following terms related to uterus.

1. Zodiacs, the ascendant and the sign that falls in fifth house, the sign in which Jupiter is placed, and the signs in which Sun and Moon are placed. This information is necessary to assess the actual constitution of uterus; function and malfunction and diseases associated with it.

2. Following are considered as male signs; all odd numbered signs like Aries, Gemini, Leo, Libra, Sagittarius and Aquarius are called as male signs or male zodiacs. Even numbered signs like Taurus, Cancer, Virgo, Scorpio, Capricorn, and Pisces are referred to as female signs or zodiacs.

3. Cancer, Scorpio and Pisces are known to give birth to more than two children; Libra, Capricorn, Aquarius gives birth to one or two kids. Whilst Aries, Leo, Sagittarius and Gemini are known as infertile zodiacs. Gemini, Sagittarius and Pisces are likely to give birth to twins.

4. Leo is normally known to cause major reasons of infertility; so also, if lord of fifth cusp is placed in Leo causes infertility.

5. Retrograde lord of fifth house with Jupiter placed afflicted with Mars, Saturn or Uranus make native suffer from infertility and even after using latest modern technologies native cannot give birth to child.

6. In Aries, Gemini, Leo and Sagittarius it is observed that the native certainly suffers from Pelvic Inflammation Disease that may lead to permanent infertility.

7.  It is noticed that if Uranus, Neptune, Ketu or Saturn placed in fifth cusp from ascendant and lord of fifth house occupies twelfth cusp intra uterine fibroids are formed.

Further while considering Uterine health we also must consider the significance of planets for instance Jupiter, Venus are known to give disease free Uterus or rising Moon in birth chart, Mercury are also if not afflicted help to keep uterus healthy. Whilst Sun, Mars, Saturn, Rahu, Ketu and Uranus, are known to cause many functional and structural disorders of uterus are required to be studied to find the possible health issues of uterus. Jupiter being main signification of fifth house if not afflicted or under aspect of malefic planet gives uterus. The significator of sixth house like Saturn or Mars if occupy fifth cusp or aspect fifth house or lord of fifth house are found to produce many infectious diseases of uterus.

Here we must not forget to understand the effect of constellation. For instance, if lord of fifth house or Jupiter occupy Ashlesha, Mula, or Kritikaun warranted growth like PCOD, or polyps, or Cysts; may also cause growth of fibroids.

As we have seen fifth house is major cusp related to uterine disorders the relation of fifth cusp with other can be clarified if we study it from ascendant.

1.  First cusp/ ascendant implies total health physical and mental health.
2.  Second cusp denotes family expansion or extinction.
3.  Fourth cusp denotes happiness on account of family and children.
4.  Fifth house denotes the uterine disorders and fertility.
5.  Seventh house indicates the health of primary reproductive organs and functional disorders of secondary reproductive organs.
6.  Eighth house is concerned with structural and functional disorders of secondary reproductive organs of female.
7.  Ninth house is concerned with the health of newborn and fetus. This also indicates fertility disorders of the infants that may occur in future.
8.  Tenth house denotes infections or of structural disorders of secondary reproductive organs.
9.  Eleventh cusp indicates functional disorders of both primary and secondary reproductive organs.
10. Twelfth cusp indicates either repeated abortions or premature death of the infants.

Certain observations which were noticed during analysis of various horoscopes are summarized here.

1. Any malefic present in fifth cusp normally gives structural disorders of uterus or hormonal problems; whilst planets like Venus, Jupiter and Mercury indicates healthy function of secondary reproductive organs.

2. If fifth house is hemmed in between malefic planets produces functional disorders of uterus like metrorrhagia, amenorrhea etc.

3. If lord of 1st, 4th 7th 10th or eleventh cusp occupy fifth house it is noticed that there are no functional or structural disorders present.

4. If fifth house is occupied by lord of sixth house or eighth house or twelfth house, then structural disorders of uterus are observed like growth of adhesions intra uterine or fibroids.

5. If lord of fifth house is placed in sixth house or eighth house or twelfth house or is afflicted with lord of any of these cusps produces inflammatory diseases of uterus.

6. If lord of fifth cusp is placed in tenth, or twelfth or fourth cusp causes functional disorders of uterus which normally are difficult to diagnose. So also, especially in tenth cusp and fourth cusp it is noticed that repeated abortion occurs specifically in first trimester.

7. If lord of fifth house is retrograde or afflicted with Uranus, Rahu, or ketu affect the growth of fetus that produces either spastic child or premature birth with severe health issues of infant health.

8. If lord of fifth house is placed in twelfth house afflicted with Rahu, Ketu, Mars, *or Uranus gives complex health disorders of infant with short life.*

9. If Sun occupies fifth house and any malefic in sign Leo causes repeated abortions due to malnutrition syndrome of mother.

10. So also, if fifth house is occupied by Moon being lord of sixth house causes repeated abortions due to malnutrition of mother especially when Saturn occupies eleventh cusp. This is typically marked by absence of cardiac activity not observed in infant during first few weeks of pregnancy.

11. If Mars occupies fifth cusp and is afflicted with Ketu or Uranus certainly gives repeated abortions as also if Saturn aspects Mars from third house or eleventh house produces physically challenged fetus that may or may not survive after birth.

12. Saturn if occupies fifth house afflicted with Uranus or Rahu causes malfunctioning of ovaries and often growth of intra uterine fibroids.

Saturn with Mars causes congenital nervous system disorders and often the newborn shall have short life.

13. Saturn Neptune conjoin in fifth house causes pelvic inflammation disease or dysfunctional bleeding. If Saturn conjoins with Neptune and under aspect of Uranus ectopic pregnancy is observed.

14. Uranus if occupies fifth house causes congenital structural or functional disordersin infant. So also, it produces severe pains during regular menstruation.

15. Often it is observed that Uranus and Neptune conjoined with any planet in fifth cusp causes severe infection of uterine canal or give rise to permanent infertility or may also cause leading to formation of repeated mutations in intra uterine layer causing cancerous growth.

16. Uranus occupied in fifth house and if native is suffering from PTSD (Post Traumatic stress Disorder) gives birth to mentally challenged child; so also, Uranus causes dysfunctional bleeding during pregnancy period that finally lead to abortion.

17. If Rahu occupies fifth cusp produces genetic disorders and sometimes birth to spastic child or irreversible Autism in child.

18. If any malefic planet present in tenth house or eighth cusp or twelfth cusp or fourth cusp is observed to cause caesarian for childbirth and gives congenital heart disorders in child.

19. If lord of fifth cusp occupies twelfth cusp and is afflicted with any malefic the native gives birth to psychologically challenged child or may be sometimes dumb and deaf child.

20. If Mars occupies eighth cusp and Moon be placed in sixth or seventh cusp gives recurring infectious diseases of uterus and uterine canal or urogenital tract and specifically infection of cervix.

21. If Moon is placed in twelfth cusp with any malefic and Mars be placed in sixth or eighth cusp causes irregular menstruation cycle and disturbed ovulation cycle.

22. If Neptune occupies fifth house and Mars placed in sixth house with Saturn placed in eleventh cusp gives heavy and prolonged flow during menstruation. In near menopausal period it is likely to produce carcinoma of cervix that may get spread to uterus.

23. If Saturn and Uranus occupy twelfth cusp the newborn may suffer from squint or other serious eye problems. If Saturn conjoins with Neptune or

Mars repeated miscarriages or abortions in first few weeks of pregnancy occur or premature birth of child is noticed.

24. If lord of twelfth cusp occupies fifth cusp causes severe pains during menstruation and produce prolonged painful back.

25. If lord of fifth cusp conjoins lord of twelfth cusp anywhere in birth chart gives Amenorrhea and sometimes oligomenorrhea or may lead to undiagnosed infertility.

26. If lord of twelfth cusp conjoins Jupiter in sixth, eighth, tenth, or twelfth cusp causes severe pain during and before menstruation and affect overall growth of body. In fourth house it causes folic acid deficiency syndrome or severe Anemia.

27. Any malefic present in fourth house normally gives prolonged infertility due to some or other functional disorders associated with uterus and ovaries. If Saturn occupies fourth house and Jupiter is placed in ascendant causes infertility due to obesity or blocked fallopian tubes.

28. Ketu or Uranus present in tenth house with fifth house occupied Mars is observed to produce health issues in newborn.

29. Saturn and Neptune if conjoined in eleventh house gives growth of polyps or cysts in ovaries; so also, if Saturn conjoins with Uranus in eleventh house severe pelvic inflammation disease which may lead to permanent infertility is noticed.

30. If Sun occupies eighth cusp and any malefic present in seventh house with Ketu in fifth cusp certainly produces leucorrhea and frequent infection of uterine canal. So also, it leads to blockages of fallopian tubes.

31. If Sun is afflicted with Rahu in seventh house and any malefic present in eighth cusp gives repeated abortions or birth to dead child. If only Rahu occupies seventh house conjoined with Sun causes serious blood related disorders in newborn infant.

32. If any malefic present in ascendant with Uranus in fifth house gives serious disorders related to ovulation and hormonal balance.

33. If Rahu be placed in fifth cusp, Mars in second house and Saturn in eighth house produce repeated infections of urogenital tract and uterine canal that may lead to infertility.

34. If Sun is placed in fifth cusp and Mars in seventh with Saturn in third house causes cancerous growth in uterus leading to hysterectomy.

35. If Mars is placed in fifth house Sun occupies eleventh cusp and Saturn being present in eighth house produces hormonal disorders and cranky behavior of the native.

36. If Saturn occupies fifth house and Sun is afflicted with Rahu in eleventh house produces infertility due to structural disorders in uterus.

37. If Uranus occupies fifth house and lord of fifth house is Mercury afflicted with Neptune the newborn may develop epileptic attacks.

38. If Saturn present in fifth house and Mars occupies eleventh house newborn may suffer from cerebral palsy.

39. If Mars occupies second cusp and Uranus is placed in fifth house or Sun occupies fifth house and Saturn is placed in eighth cusp causes Adenomyosis i.e. ectopic growth of endometrial tissue within the myometrium.

40. If Jupiter afflicted with Ketu in fifth house and Mars placed in twelfth house afflicted with Uranus Endometritis infection in uterine cavity or malformations including uterine didelphys bicomuate or septate uterus is observed.

41. Retrograde Jupiter in fifth house specifically in sign Leo causes Hematometra i.e. accumulation of blood in Uterine cavity.

42. Jupiter if afflicted with Neptune in fifth cusp, Mars in eighth house, Afflicted Moon in twelfth cusp is observed to give myometritis i.e. severe inflammation of muscular uterine wall.

# Chapter 3

# Lords and Uterine Diseases

So far, we have seen various combinations of planes and cusps that produce different disorders of the Uterus and we have studied the effects of those combinations on uterine function and on structural disorders. It is noteworthy here that though it appears difficult to correlate the specific disorder with specific planetary combination, it is very much possible to locate the basic cause which requires to be diagnosed or to be observed in detail. In human being it is though appears next to impossible to have prolonged observation, but it is certainly possible to take remedial actions in time and to bring the disorder in control.

In this chapter we can see how to understand and correlate specific problem with specific planetary combination or the direction of our mode of treatment and tools to be used for diagnosis can be charted out in specific way.

There are various tools and techniques are used to study the exact onset of the disease and diagnostic tests to arrive at specific problem such as anti-Mullerianhormone test may be conducted when Saturn and Ketu are present in fifth house. This is also applicable when Mars is placed in eighth house and Moon occupies seventh house.

If the relation of planets with the diseases or disorder is studied, we may find the tabulated results as mentioned herewith.

There are total of 11 sub clauses we can divide to understand this relation and here we can find out the causes, symptoms and involvement of planetary status in birth chart as detailed bellow.

1.  **Urinary Tract Infections**

    This is commonly called as UTI and considered major contributor to most of the problems related to disorders and diseases of Uterus. This is caused by Fungi, Virus, and Bacteria; of these Bacterial infections are most common. UTI can occur at any age group and any region of urinary tract; this condition may be extremely painful and can affect urethras, genital tract and bladder. Few common symptoms may include

    i.    Foul smell of urine,

    ii.   Cloudy, dark or bloody urine,

    iii.  A frequent urge to urinate,

    iv.   Pain or burning sensation while urinating,

    v.    Pressure or cramp in back or lower abdomen,

    vi.   Muscle aches,

    vii.  Fatigue,

    viii. Vomiting,

    ix.   Nausea,

    x.    Pelvic pain, pain in center of pelvis, and area around pubic zone,

    xi.   Fever or chills.

    Normally following conditions may increase risk of UTI

    a.    Difficulty in emptying bladder completely,

    b.    Diabetes,

    c.    A weak immune system,

    d.    Certain conditions that obstruct urinary tract,

    e.    Using contraceptive diaphragm that is coated with spermicidal.

    When in birth chart of the women suffering from these disorders, we find following combinations well spelled and almost repeated in every birth chart of the women.

    i.    Mainly it is observed that fifth house is hemmed in between malefic in all charts.

    ii.   It was noticed that lord of fifth house is placed in sixth cusp and is afflicted with Uranus.

    iii.  Mars found to have occupied fifth house afflicted with Ketu or Uranus.

    iv.   It was also observed that Neptune placed in fifth cusp conjoined with Saturn and is under aspect of Mars.

**2.  Infertility in women**

This was independently studied, and it was interesting to note that following factors were observed in almost all the cases we have studied.

i.    Premature ovarian failure.

ii.   Polycystic ovarian syndrome,

iii.  Hyperprolactenemia,

iv.   Poor egg quality,

v.    Overactive thyroid gland,

vi.   Underactive thyroid gland,

vii.  Other chronic conditions such as cancer.

Apart from these some structural disorders are also responsible for infertility like blockages in fallopian tubes. Fallopian tubes are pathways where the egg travels from ovary reaching to the uterus where the egg grows into zygote. If something abnormal or due to adhesions in fallopian tubes or uterus woman may not be able to conceive. Factors responsible for the blockages are,

i.    Blocked fallopian tubes due to obesity or PID.

ii.   Surgery,

iii.  Sub mucosal fibroid,

iv.   Endometriosis,

v.    Previous sterilization treatment,

vi.   Medications such as Non-Steroidal Anti-inflammatory drugs,

vii.  Chemotherapy,

viii. Radiation therapy of any part near reproductive system,

ix.   Consumption of Illegal drugs such as marijuana, cocaine.

The major planetary combinations found that trigger these

a.    If Mars occupies eighth cusp and Moon is placed in seventh cusp with Saturn and Uranus present in eleventh house is observed to produce structural obstructive disorders.

b.    If Jupiter occupies ascendant in any sign and Mars is placed in fifth house with Saturn in ninth cusp makes native voracious eater and gives obesity and this obesity causes blockages of Fallopian tubes due to collection of fat tissue around.

c.    In case Mars is occupied in fifth cusp and Sun present in eleventh cusp with Saturn in eighth cusp gives adhesions in Fallopian tubes.

### 3. Menstrual disorders

Menstruation disorders range from uncomfortable symptoms leading up to period to more serious conditions such as menstruation being too heavy or light, irregular periods or even complete absence of cycle. Major common menstruation disorders causes, symptoms and planetary relation is briefed as bellow.

i. Premenstrual syndrome or PMS tends to occur a week or two before period starts and symptoms associated are irritability, fatigue, cramps, breast soreness, headache, back ache, Acne, diarrhea, bloating, insomnia, anxiety, depression, feeling stressed, food craving, and emotional mood swing. PMS symptoms could vary each month and symptoms go away with period starts.

ii. Heavy periods i.e. bleeding is heavier than usual, may experience extended periods even beyond 5-7 days. The cause is mainly hormonal level imbalance especially estrogen and progesterone. Also changes in diet, exercise, vaginal infections, hypothyroidism, fibroids, puberty and inflammation of cervix.

iii. Painful periods some physical pain and cramp are common during beginning of periods however some women experience severe pain throughout their period. The menstrual pain is due to underlying medical condition such as fibroids, endometriosis and pelvic inflammatory disease.

iv. Missing periods or Amenorrhea can be classified in two types,

- Primary Amenorrhea, in this case female does not get her first period till her age of 16 years and it is referred to as primary Amenorrhea.

- Secondary Amenorrhea in this case grown up woman miss periods for six months or more consecutively and causes vary for adults and teenagers, it could be because sudden weight gain or weight loss. This also may be due to anorexia, discontinuation of birth control pills, ovarian cyst, and overactive thyroid gland, in adult it could be due to pregnancy, premature ovarian failure, pelvic inflammation disease, menopause, or discontinuing birth control pills.

The planetary disposition responsible for menstruation disorders is given herewith for further study and confirmation.

i.    If lord of twelfth house occupies fifth cusp and any malefic present in eleventh house causes functional disorders such as menstrual disorders.

ii.   If Saturn occupies fifth house with Uranus and Mars is placed in sixth house hormonal disorders like Amenorrhea, Metrorrhagia, dysfunctional bleeding occurs.

iii.  If Saturn is afflicted with Neptune in fifth house and Mars placed in eighth cusp certainly gives Pelvic Inflammation Disorder.

iv.   If any malefic present in tenth house and Mars occupies fifth house afflicted with Uranus causes menstrual disorders.

v.    If Moon placed in twelfth house and any malefic with Mars occupies eighth cusp gives prolonged periods with heavy discharge.

4.  **Miscarriages** medically it is known as spontaneous abortion or loss of pregnancy and generally occurs in first 13 weeks of pregnancy. It accompanies several difficult moments specifically related to the psychological health of the woman. There are different types of miscarriages each having different treatments and planetary disposition that causes it to happen. There are several reasons of abortion and exact cause cannot be identified but can be defined with the help of horoscope or birth chart of woman.

The most common cause of miscarriage during first trimester of pregnancy is chromosomal abnormalities which mean that something is not right with baby's chromosomes; most often chromosomal abnormality is caused by diseased sperm or cell or a problem when zygote went through process of divisions and may also include one or many of following causes.

i.    Hormonal disorders, maternal health, infections.

ii.   Lifestyle which includes smoking, malnutrition, excessive caffeine, drug abuse or exposure to toxic substances or radiation.

iii.  Maternal trauma,

iv.   Uterine abnormalities,

The major signs or symptoms include

i.    Spotting or bleeding,

ii.   Abdominal pains.

The major causes that increases risk of miscarriage include

i. Age which is significant factor that plays a role in conceiving elder woman; are more likely to conceive baby with chromosomal abnormalities resulting into miscarriage.

ii. Chronic diseases or disorders like uncontrolled diabetes, or certaininherited blood clotting disorders or hormonal disorders, autoimmune diseases.

iii. History of miscarriages; if a woman has experienced two or more miscarriages in a row increases risk of further miscarriage.

iv. Uterine or cervical problems; that have certain congenital abnormalities, a weak or abnormally short cervix or severe uterine adhesions are often likely to experience miscarriage.

v. A history of congenital disabilities of genetic problems; if woman or partner or their close relatives have genetic abnormalities or woman from their close relation have given a birth to child with congenital abnormalities are at higher risk of miscarriage.

vi. Addictions like smoking, drinking alcohol, drug use, such as cocaine, high level of caffeine also causes miscarriage.

The responsible planetary disposition in birth chart of woman can be summarized as given herewith.

i. If Sun is afflicted with Rahu in seventh house with any malefic present in eighth cusp gives repeated miscarriages.

ii. If lord of twelfth house conjoins Jupiter in sixth or eighth or tenth or twelfth house and Mars occupies sixth cusp causes repeated abortions.

iii. If Uranus occupies fifth cusp and woman is suffering from PTSD (Post Traumatic Stress Disorder) gives dysfunctional bleeding during pregnancy that leads to miscarriage.

iv. Saturn and Neptune conjoin in fifth cusp may give ectopic pregnancy that result in miscarriage.

v. If Mars occupies fifth house and is afflicted with Ketu or Uranus certainly gives abortions.

vi. If Sun occupies fifth house, then repeated abortions are caused due to various functional disorders.

vii. If Moon is placed in fifth cusp being lord of sixth house causes repeated abortions and especially when at the same time Saturn is placed in eleventh house produces miscarriage or abortion due to absence of cardiac activities in fetus during first few weeks of pregnancy.

viii. If lord of fifth house is placed in tenth cusp or twelfth cusp or fourth house produces functional disorders which are difficult to diagnose and especially if it is tenth house repeated miscarriages are noticed.

## 5. Low Amniotic Fluid

Amniotic fluid is baby's life support system that protects the baby and assists in development of muscles, lungs, limbs and digestive system. This fluid is produced soon after amniotic sac is formed i.e. about within 12 days of post conception. It is first made up of water provided by mother and by about 20 weeks the fetal urine becomes primary substance; in second trimester baby will begin breathing and swallowing the amniotic fluid. Normally low amniotic fluid or oligohydramnios can occur mostly during last trimester of pregnancy. The major causes for low amniotic fluid can be summarized as follows.

i.     Congenital disabilities which include development of kidneys or urinary tract.
ii.    Leaking or rupture of membranes,
iii.   Problems with placenta,
iv.    Postdate pregnancy,
v.     Maternal complications such as hypertension during pregnancy, preeclampsia, maternal dehydration, diabetes and chronic hypoxia.

This condition is generally observed when following planetary disposition is noticed.

a.     If lord of fifth house is retrograde and afflicted with Uranus or Neptune and eighth cusp is occupied by Mars, then low amniotic fluid or rupture of membrane or leaking of amniotic fluid is observed.
b.     If fifth house is occupied by lord of eighth cusp and Saturn or Uranus occupies eleventh house placental problems or occurred.
c.     If lord of fifth cusp is placed in fourth cusp and is under aspect of any malefic from tenth house tends to give severe dehydration of mother and likely to produce preeclampsia.
d.     If any malefic present in tenth cusp or eighth house tends to cause low amniotic fluid syndrome and caesarian for childbirth.

6. **Diabetes in pregnancy**

   Diabetes is critical metabolic disorder in which either Beta cells in pancreas do produce less Insulin or produce no insulin. Also, if released insulin does not help cell absorb serum glucose required for their growth metabolism or activities involving energy release like dephosphorylation of ATP into ADP.

   There are two main types of diabetes,

   i. Type-1 diabetes this kind of diabetes is an autoimmune disorder and needs regular use of insulin. The symptoms may include constant hunger, weight loss, increased thirst, frequent urination, blurred vision and fatigue.

   ii. Type-2 diabetes is most common form often associated with age, family history, obesity, physical inactivity and previous history of gestational diabetes. The symptoms include infection of bladder, or kidney, increased thirst, frequent urination, fatigue, constant hunger. There are few potentially health risk for the infant when mother has diabetes.

   a. Macrosomia- in this condition baby grows too large due to excess amount of insulin that crosses through placenta. Large baby can cause difficulty in vaginal delivery and increases risk of injury to baby during process of birth.

   b. Hypoglycaemia also known as low blood sugar level and this condition can develop soon after birth of baby due to high levels insulin. Controlling blood sugar can help lower the risk of this condition for baby.

   c. Jaundice a yellowish discoloration of the eyes and skin can sometimes be attributed to diabetes in pregnancy.

   The astrological correlation of this pregnancy diabetes can easily be detected in birth chart. Some of following planetary combinations can be considered as major indicators of this condition in pregnancy.

   i. If Mars occupies fifth house and Venus is placed in eighth cusp in fixed sign like Gemini may produce pregnancy diabetes.

   ii. If Uranus occupied in fifth house and Saturn placed in eleventh house with Venus placed in sixth cusp likely to cause pregnancy diabetes and in such cases the diabetes is observed to be genetically transmitted from mother or father.

iii. If lord of fifth house is placed in twelfth cusp and Venus occupies sixth cusp with Saturn being placed in fourth cusp then native is certain to suffer from pregnancy diabetes which generally gets vanished after childbirth.

iv. If Saturn afflicted with Neptune in eleventh cusp and Mars occupies afflicted with Uranus in fifth cusp so also Venus is placed in eighth house is likely to cause Type 1 diabetes that exists prior to conception and aggravates during pregnancy.

v. If Neptune occupies fifth cusp and Venus afflicted with Mars placed in eighth house gives birth to large baby and likely to cause injury to baby while labour.

vi. If Moon is placed in twelfth cusp with Mars in moving sign in fifth house and Venus occupies sixth cusp the native is certain to give birth to bay who suffers from Jaundice after birth.

vii. If Saturn occupies fifth house, Mars is placed in second cusp with Venus in eighth cusp causes Hypoglycemia and sometimes hypoxia that leads to premature birth of child.

7. **Hypertension in pregnancy** commonly known as high blood pressure is one of the most common problems that is encountered during pregnancy and is defined as Blood pressure higher than 140/90 mm of mercury. This condition during pregnancy is not always dangerous but can sometimes causes serious complications for both mother and unborn baby. Following are types of pregnancy related hypertension conditions.

i. Chronic hypertension this condition is referred to as pre-existing hypertension before woman gets pregnant. Sometimes hypertension that occurs within first 20 weeks of pregnancy is also referred to as chronic hypertension. And often treated with blood pressure medications.

ii. Gestational hypertension this kind of hypertension is usually developed after 20 weeks of pregnancy and often resolves after birth of child. The most common complication that gestational hypertension brings along is induced labor.

iii. Chronic hypertension with superimposed preeclampsia, in this condition along with preexisting high blood pressure experiences protein in the urine or additional complications as the pregnancy progresses.

The major causes of hypertension in pregnancy can be summarized as bellow.

a.  Overweight or obesity,

b.  Absence of physical activity or exercises.

c.  Age,

d.  First time pregnancy,

e.  Carrying more than one child,

f.  Family history of hypertension in pregnancy.

g.  Smoking,

h.  Alcohol consumption,

i.  Assistive technology used for pregnancy such as IVF.

Planetary disposition for pregnancy hypertension can be briefed as given herewith.

i.  If sign Aquarius falls in fourth cusp and Mars occupies it with Moon occupies eleventh house and is under aspect of Saturn from fifth house causes pregnancy blood pressure which normally creates complications in last trimester of pregnancy.

ii.  If Mars occupies Leo in fifth cusp and Mercury is placed in Cancer certainly causes pregnancy hypertension. This normally is found preexisting hypertension.

iii.  If Sun occupies Cancer in fourth cusp and Saturn placed in tenth house with Neptune conjoins with Mars in fifth cusp gives pregnancy blood pressure that gets recovered as soon as the birth of child.

iv.  If Mercury occupies Aquarius in fourth house and Sun afflicted with Ketu placed in fifth cusp causes pregnancy hypertension.

v.  If Mars placed in Cancer in fifth house and

Saturn occupies sixth house with Sun placed in eighth cusp causes pregnancy hypertension that vanishes away with childbirth.

8.  **Cervical cancer** occurs when normal cells of cervix grow abnormally; cervix is being lower part of uterus the occurrence of this type of cancer is more than other types of cancer. It is caused by Human Papilloma Virus or HPV which is sexually transmitted from one person to another and includes major symptoms

i.  Abnormal vaginal bleeding,

ii.  Pain during intercourse,

iii.    Abnormal vaginal discharge,

iv.    Pain in pelvic or lower belly.

Major planetary combinations are summed up bellow.

a.    If Saturn is occupied in fifth cusp with Sun in eighth house afflicted with Ketu, and if Mars present in eleventh cusp causes repeated mutations of cells in cervix that leads to cancer ultimately.

b.    If Mars occupies sixth cusp in Virgo afflicted with Neptune and Saturn occupies fifth cusp with Uranus present in eleventh house certainly leads to cancerous growth in cervix or Uterus.

c.    If Venus afflicted with Uranus placed in Scorpio in eighth cusp and Saturn present in eleventh house with sign Aquarius likely to give abnormal growth of cells in cervix that causes cancer.

9.    **Breast cancer,** this type of cancer is occurred when breast cells grow abnormally producing lump or lumps in breast tissues. These cells tend to form hard tumor which can be felt or seen in X ray screening. This may spread into surrounding areas of body and is generally observed to be malignant. The brief causes of this type of cancer can be summed up as,

i.    Advancing age, women over 50 years of age,

ii.    Family history of breast cancer,

iii.    Presence of benign tumors in breast,

iv.    Over exposure to hormone estrogen,

The major symptoms noticed are

a.    Skin irritation or dimpling,

b.    Nipples turning inwards,

c.    Nipples discharge fluid other than milk,

d.    Breast or nipple pain,

e.    Scaling, thickening, or redness of nipple or breast.

Sometimes it spreads into lymph nodes around the collar bone, and cause swelling; even swollen lymph nodes indicate malignant tumor in breast. The major planetary disposition noticed is as briefed bellow,

1.    Saturn occupies third house afflicted with Rahu and Mars is placed in fifth cusp under aspect of Uranus from eleventh house generally

    indicated family history of breast cancer and native is also likely to suffer from breast cancer.

2. If lord of eighth cusp is associated with Neptune and Mars occupies fifth house afflicted with Saturn induces hormonal disorders that in latter stage after menopause give cancerous growth in breast; this is normally seen irrecoverable.

3. If Jupiter conjuncts with Rahu or Mars in watery sign especially in twelfth house and Mercury occupies fifth house afflicted with Saturn causes growth of malignant tumors in breast.

4. If Mars is placed in fifth cusp with sign Libra and Moon occupies eighth cusp conjoined with lord of seventh house is certain to give breast cancer after 50 years of age.

10. **Uterine cancer,** this is occurring when uncontrolled growth of endometrial wall of uterus which begins with abnormal growth of cells is noticed. This comprises uterine tissues, or forms of muscles of other tissues of uterus. Common symptoms include abnormal vaginal bleeding, or fluid discharge, the occurrence of pain after urination, or after sexual intercourse, or pelvic pain. While mainly it affects women, who have not had pregnancy in life; it can also affect women who have experienced early menstruation, or who have already undergone menopause. To ascertain that woman, have uterine cancer it is imperative that she is aware of the symptoms that indicate this condition. Major symptoms which can be noticed may include,

a. Abnormal dysfunctional vaginal bleeding,

b. Abnormal fluid discharge sometimes watery or sometimes blood tinged.

c. Vaginal bleeding after menopause,

d. Pelvic pain.

There are two main types occurred in uterine cancer and are i) Endometrial cancer which develops in the lining of uterus and is most common that accounts for almost 95% of uterine cancer. ii) Uterine sarcoma which is rare type and generally occur in muscles or tissues of uterus or tissues which hold it up in position. Once uterine cancer is diagnosed the extent can be classified into stages I to IV as detailed bellow:

i.   This stage where cancerous growth is detected only in uterus with possible growth in the glands of cervix.

ii.  The growth of cancerous cells is found in the body of uterus and into the supporting connective tissues of cervix called cervical stroma.

iii. The growth of cancerous cells is found spread beyond uterus and may affect lymph nodes and pelvic area.

iv.  In this stage growth of cancer is found to have propagated into other areas affecting bladder, rectum and sometimes also found to have occurred in bones, omentum or lungs.

The classic planetary disposition noticed was

1.   If Venus occupies ascendant with sign Sagittarius and afflicted with Uranus, the Mars conjoins Saturn in fifth house and Neptune occupies eighth cusp conjoined with Jupiter the uterine cancer is noticed and even after hysterectomy was found to have reoccurred leading to confirm death.

2.   If Mars conjoins Mercury in fifth house with sign Aquarius and Sun occupies eighth cusp afflicting with Ketu or Uranus is noticed to have produced uterine cancer; in this condition normally the diagnosis is confirmed when cancer in its advanced stage and becomes incurable.

3.   If Moon conjoins Mars in fifth house with sign Libra and Venus occupies seventh house afflicted with Saturn and Uranus found to have caused cancer of cervix which was recovered after surgical procedure.

4.   If Sun occupies ascendant in sign Aquarius and Saturn is placed in seventh house afflicted with Uranus and Jupiter occupied in fourth or sixth cusp certainly causes uterine cancer which becomes complicated to treat.

5.   If Sun is placed in fifth house with sign Virgo and afflicted with Neptune with Saturn occupies eighth cusp and Mars in ascendant gives uterine cancer after menopause.

6.   If Sun is placed in ascendant with sign Capricorn and Mars occupies fifth house afflicted with Uranus with Ketu placed in tenth cusp certainly causes cancer of cervix to occur which over period gets spread into adjoining areas.

7.   If Rahu occupies fifth house with sign Scorpio and Mars placed in eleventh house afflicted with Uranus causes Pelvic Inflammation Disorder which potentially develops into uterine cancer and gives complications.

8.   If Sun is placed in tenth house with sign Capricorn afflicted with Rahu and Mars is placed in fourth house conjoined with Ketu causes Sarcoma of uterine wall or muscles.

11. **Menopause** this is particularly important phase in woman's life when menstrual periods stop and marks the end of fertile period. It is said to occur within twelve months of last menstrual period is noticed. In this phase ovaries stop producing estrogen and progesterone hormones essential for reproduction. This phase leads to major changes called menopausal symptoms and often requires to be clinically attended.

a.   Vaginal dryness, sometimes irritation and itching,
b.   Disturbed sleep,
c.   Mood swing,
d.   Trouble trying focus,
e.   Weight gain with slowed metabolism,
f.   Irregular periods,
g.   Hot flashes,
h.   Night sweats,
i.   Hair loss, or thinning of hairs,
j.   Loss of feeling of breast full,

Being this is natural phenomena no planetary disposition can be correlated, whilst associated disorders like increase in hypertension or obesity are required to be studied as usual.

# Chapter 4

# Examples of Uterine Infection

After considering these disorders and diseases of uterus and related organs we need to understand their correlation with planetary disposition as discussed earlier and this can be well explained by the study of few practical examples. We here can study the various cases with their planetary disposition and actual correlation to understand the individual effect of planes.

1.  Urinary tract infection This normally occurs when fifth house is hemmed between malefic or other various combinations as discussed before.

Case No. 001/o ab
Native born on 26ᵗʰ July 1984 at 01:30 hrs. In Aurangabad
Lat. 019:48N Long. 075:19

This is a classical case which if we study can understand the occurrence of uterine and urinary tract infection. This is Taurus ascendant and Rahu and the lord of ascendant is placed in third cusp with sign Cancer and conjoined with Sun. The Moon is placed in second cusp with sign Gemini, the lord of second cusp Mercury is occupied in fourth cusp with sign Leo. The lord of seventh cusp and twelfth cusp Mars is placed in sixth cusp with sign Venus, Mars is afflicted with Saturn which is lord of ninth and eleventh cusp. Saturn aspects ascendant and lord of seventh cusp Venus and Sun. Ketu is placed in seventh cusp conjoined with Uranus aspects ascendant. Jupiter lord of eighth and eleventh cusp is placed in eighth cusp afflicted with Neptune. In this case first we can observe Mars is significator of Blood and Saturn is significator of obstruction or chronic type of inflammation and infection and both are conjoined in sixth house indicating the repetitive occurrence of infection and so also Venus which is significator of reproductive organ and is under aspect of Saturn indicating inflammation of reproductive organ. Another fact we can observe in this case is Jupiter which is causative of structural disorder is also under aspect of Saturn and as such creates the disorder of epithelial layers of vaginal vault and urinary tract. Further the lord of seventh house Mars occupied in sixth house with sign Venus which again is causative of reproductive organ is afflicted in malefic house and occupied by Mars conjoined with Saturn indicates the inflammation of the organ. So also, it is noticed in this birth chart that Sun the significator of functional disorder is occupied in Cancer and is under aspect of Saturn gives functional disorder as the immunity in this specific organ is reduced. Further the significator of cellular growth and hormonal function is Moon which is placed in second house with sign Gemini and is under aspect of Neptune and Ketu as such is responsible for inflammatory disorder of lining of urinary tract causing infection. If the planetary disposition is seen it can be clear that in this case first medication for increase in immunity is required to be administered and simultaneously the medication for infection and inflammation can be given.

The planetary disposition can be studied in the chart given as under.

| Planet | Zodiac | Degrees | Lord zodiac | Star lord | Sub lord |
|---|---|---|---|---|---|
| Sun | Cancer | 069:23:21 | Moon | Sat | Ven |
| Moon | Gemini | 034:14:17 | Mercury | Mar | Ven |
| Mars | Libra | 175:43:18 | Venus | Jupiter | Mer |
| Mercury | Leo | 095:49:15 | Sun | Ketu | Rah |
| Jupiter | Sagitta | 221:20:20 | Jupiter | Ketu | Sat |
| Venus | Cancer | 080:22:55 | Moon | Merc. | Ven |
| Saturn | Libra | 166:11:29 | Venus | Rahu | Ven |
| Rahu | Taurus | 009:56:30 | Venus | Sun | Ven |
| Ketu | Scorpio | 189:56:30 | Mars | Sat | Ven |
| Uranus | Scorpio | 196:07:19 | Mars | Sat | Jup |
| Neptune | Sagitta. | 215:32:42 | Jupiter | Ketu | Mar |

If according to KP system, we observe it again we find that

| Cusp | Sign in cusp | Lord of cusp | Star Lord | Sub lord |
|---|---|---|---|---|
| 01 | Taurus | Venus | Sun | Mercury |
| 02 | Gemini | Mercury | Mars | Mercury |
| 03 | Gemini | Mercury | Jupiter | Venus |
| 04 | Cancer | Moon | Mercury | Moon |
| 05 | Leo | Sun | Venus | Saturn |
| 06 | Virgo | Mercury | Mars | Saturn |
| 07 | Scorpio | Mars | Saturn | Saturn |
| 08 | Sagittarius | Jupiter | Ketu | Venus |
| 09 | Sagittarius | Jupiter | Venus | Ketu |
| 10 | Capricorn | Saturn | Moon | Sun |
| 11 | Aquarius | Saturn | Jupiter | Saturn |
| 12 | Pisces | Jupiter | Mercury | Saturn |

In this chart also it is clear that lord of sixth house Mars is placed in sixth house with sub lord of twelfth cusp and star lord of sixth cusp Saturn which aggravates the infection of urinary tract. Further star lord of eighth cusp Ketu is placed in seventh house and as such afflicted the seventh house which is significator of reproductive tract causing the inflammation. So also, the Star lord of ascendant is under aspect of Saturn which is star lord of sixth cusp and sub lord of twelfth cusp. Further sub lord of eighth cusp Venus conjoins Sun in third house which is significator of reproductive system and under aspect of Saturn causes the occurrence of repeated infection of urinary tract and reproductive system tract.

As such by applying any system of Astrological prediction it is easy to understand the probable disorder or disease that is likely to occur.

Case No. 002/vj

The native born on 25th May 1990 at 11:45 hrs. In Jalgaon.

Latitude 021:06N Longitude 075:36E

This is Leo ascendant chart and the lord of ascendant Sun is occupied in tenth cusp with sign Taurus conjoined with Moon. Fifth cusp is occupied by Uranus conjoined with Neptune in sign Sagittarius. Saturn is placed in sixth cusp in own sign Capricorn afflicted with Rahu. Saturn is also lord of seventh house. Mars is placed in eighth cusp with sign Pisces under aspect of Saturn. Mercury lord of second and eleventh cusp is placed in ninth house with sign Aries, Mercury is conjoined with Venus which is lord of tenth and third cusp. Jupiter lord of fifth and eighth cusp is occupied in eleventh house with sign Gemini. Ketu is placed in twelfth house with sign Cancer. Lord of twelfth cusp Moon is occupied in tenth house conjoined with Sun which is lord of ascendant this clearly indicates the reduced level of immunity which causes repeated infections. Fifth house is occupied by Uranus conjoined with another malefic planet Neptune also indicates the dryness of epithelial, mucosal lining of urinary tract that allows the growth of Fungus or Bacteria in the tract giving infection and inflammation. Lord of seventh house Saturn is placed in sixth cusp afflicted with Rahu and is under aspect of Ketu gives recurring structural disorders of the urinary and genital tract. Mars lord of fourth cusp and ninth cusp is occupied in eighth cusp causing repeated sever infection of genital tract; Mars is also under aspect of Saturn indicates inflammation of mucosal membrane of urinary and genital tract. Further lord of Virgo Mercury is placed in ninth house is under aspect of Ketu from twelfth house indicates reduced immunity of the native that causes repeated infections.

This also can be clarified by KP system. Lord of ascendant Sun is also star lord of sixth house conjoined with lord of twelfth house Moon that denotes the growth of fungus or Bacteria in the urinary tract that causes repeated infections. Star lord of eighth house Jupiter which is also star lord of twelfth cusp is placed in eleventh house, aspect fifth house thereby causing inflammatory diseases of genital tract. Sub lord of ascendant Venus which is also sub lord of eighth cusp is occupied in ninth cusp conjoined with Venus which is sub lord of eighth cusp and thus well connected with ascendant gives recurring genital tract inflammation. Again, sub lord of twelfth cusp Rahu is occupied in sixth cusp conjoined with lord of seventh cusp indicates the repeated infection of urinary tract.

In this case it is also observed that the onset of the disease occurred when Rahu mahadasha was in progress and ANTARDASHA and Pratiantardasha of Jupiter was started.

Planetary disposition of case no 002/vj is tabled herewith for reference.

| Planet | Zodiac | Degrees | Lord of Zodiac | Star lord | Sub lord |
|---|---|---|---|---|---|
| Sun | Taurus | 280:03:56 | Venus | Moon | Moon |
| Moon | Taurus | 291:02:51 | Venus | Moon | Venus. |
| Mars | Pisces | 211:50:04 | Jupiter | Jupiter | Rahu |
| Mercury | Aries | 256:41:17 | Mars | Venus | Moon |
| Jupiter | Gemini | 317:43:04 | Mercury | Rahu | Sun |
| Venus | Aries | 240:17:50 | Mars | Ketu | Ketu |
| Saturn | Capricorn | 151:17:04 | Saturn | Sun | Jupiter. |
| Rahu | Capricorn | 167:05:30 | Saturn | Moon | Saturn. |
| Ketu | Cancer | 347:05:30 | Moon | Mercur | Merc. |
| Uranus | Sagittarius | 135:11:18 | Jupiter | Venus | Venus |
| Neptune | Sagittarius | 140:27:48 | Jupiter | Venus | Jupiter. |

The KP sub lord can be found as below,

| Cusp | zodiac | Lord zodiac | Star lord | Sub lord |
|---|---|---|---|---|
| 01 | Leo | Sun | Ketu | Venus |
| 02 | Leo | Sun | Sun | Mars |
| 03 | Virgo | Mercury | Mars | Saturn |
| 04 | Scorpio | Mars | Jupiter | Mars |
| 05 | Sagittarius | Jupiter | Ketu | Venus |
| 06 | Capricorn | Saturn | Sun | Jupiter |
| 07 | Aquarius | Saturn | Mars | Mercury |
| 08 | Aquarius | Saturn | Jupiter | Venus |
| 09 | Pisces | Jupiter | Mercury | Saturn |
| 10 | Taurus | Venus | Sun | Rahu |
| 11 | Gemini | Mercury | Mars | Mercury |
| 12 | Cancer | Moon | Jupiter | Rahu |

Case No. 003/apk

The native is born on 13th December 1990 at 00:20 hrs in Mumbai/Borivili with Lat. 019:13 N, Long. 072:51E

The first look at chart clearly indicates the affliction of fifth house with Saturn, Uranus and Neptune along with afflicted Venus conjoined with Mercury. Tenth cusp is occupied which is lord of fourth and ninth house aspect Sun lord of ascendant placed in fourth cusp. Lord of fifth house and eighth house Jupiter is occupied in twelfth cusp afflicted with Ketu in sign Cancer. Lord of twelfth house Moon is placed in third house with sign Libra. In this disposition we can see firstly fifth house is afflicted indicating its vulnerability to diseases due to presence of Uranus and Neptune; further Saturn also occupies the same house indicating obstructive and inflammatory diseases of organs ruled by fifth house so also Saturn being lord of seventh house denotes the inflammatory diseases of genital tract as it is afflicted with Uranus. Venus is being significator of reproductive organs and Mercury being ruler of skin or epithelial and mucosal lining of urinary and genital tract, are severely afflicted with Saturn and Neptune causes recurring infection of urinary and genital tract. Further Uranus occupied in fifth cusp indicates mysterious infection which normally goes unnoticed for long period till it impacts the functional disorder of the organ. Particularly in this case the UTI escalates further to cause Pelvic Inflammation Disease that also gives infertility. It is significant in this case that even the lord of fifth house Jupiter is occupied in twelfth house afflicted with Ketu which reduces the immunity leading to uncontrolled infection. So also it is noticeable to observe the Moon which signifies the immunity function is also under aspect of Rahu and in quincunx with Mars causing it debilitated reduces the immunity function and as such aggravates the infection and inflammation of urinary tract and genital tract. It is also interesting to note here that lord of ascendant Sun is placed in fourth cusp with sign Scorpio and is also under aspect of Mars from tenth house gives overall reduced immunity and energy required to be active which may cause cardiac problems due to hormonal and steroidal disorders. Because of pelvic inflammation disease also called as PID repeated blockages of fallopian tubes infertility occurs.

With reference to the KP system we can see here in this case that star lord of first house Venus is occupied in fifth house afflicted with Uranus and Neptune and conjoined with star lord of eighth cusp and twelfth cusp Mercury which denotes the structural and functional disorders of urinary tract, genital tract and pelvis. Star lord of sixth cusp Mars is occupied in tenth house is in quincunx with Saturn, Uranus and Neptune indicates severe fungal or bacterial infection that becomes chronic over passage of time due to Saturn. Further it also can be noticed that sub lord of ascendant Saturn is placed fifth cusp is afflicted with Uranus and Neptune. The sub lord of twelfth house Rahu is occupied in sixth house and aspect Moon which is sub lord of eighth cusp and thus ascendant, sixth cusp and eighth cusp are well connected indicates the repeated infection and inflammation of urinary and genital tract.

This is a classic case which can be studied in different aspect by different methodologies of prediction and if correlated with actual medical diagnostic findings gives crystal clear indication of predicted structural and functional disorders of urogenital tract of the native.

The planetary disposition of case no 003/apk can be tabled as bellow.

| planet | zodiac | Degrees | Lord zodiac | Star lord | Sub lord |
| --- | --- | --- | --- | --- | --- |
| Sun | Scorpio | 116:45:07 | Mars | Mercury | Jupiter |
| Moon | Libra | 068:58:00 | Venus | Rahu | Jupiter |
| Mars | Taurus | 276:39:18 | Venus | Sun | Mercury |
| Mercury | Sagittarius | 135:54:17 | Jupiter | Venus | Sun |
| Jupiter | Cancer | 349:36:07 | Moon | Mercury | Venus |
| Venus | Sagittarius | 126:52:09 | Jupiter | Ketu | Rahu |
| Saturn | Sagittarius | 149:47:00 | Jupiter | Sun | Rahu |
| Rahu | Capricorn | 156:24:42 | Saturn | Sun | Merc |
| Ketu | Cancer | 326:24:42 | Moon | Saturn | Merc |
| Uranus | Sagittarius | 134:51:28 | Jupiter | Venus | Venus |
| Neptune | Sagittarius | 139:40:24 | Jupiter | Venus | Rahu |

According to KP system Cusp division and sub lords

| Cusp | Zodiac | Zodiac lord | Star lord | Sub lord |
| --- | --- | --- | --- | --- |
| 01 | Leo | Sun | Venus | Saturn |
| 02 | Virgo | Mercury | Moon | Sun |
| 03 | Libra | Venus | Jupiter | Saturn |
| 04 | Scorpio | Mars | Mercury | Mars |
| 05 | Sagittarius | Jupiter | Venus | Mercury |
| 06 | Capricorn | Saturn | Mars | Rahu |
| 07 | Aquarius | Saturn | Jupiter | Saturn |
| 08 | Pisces | Jupiter | Mercury | Moon |
| 09 | Aries | Mars | Venus | Saturn |
| 10 | Taurus | Venus | Mars | Mars |
| 11 | Gemini | Mercury | Jupiter | Mercury |
| 12 | Cancer | Moon | Mercury | Rahu |

Case No. 004/tvs
The native born on 24th April 1978 at 18:05 hours in Sawantwadi
Lat. 015:54 N Long. 073:48E

This is a Libra ascendant birth chart with lord of ascendant placed in eighth house with sign Taurus; also, Venus is under aspect of Neptune occupied in Scorpio. Moon is placed in ascendant afflicted with Uranus which indicates that ascendant is afflicted causing reduced immunity and vulnerability to repeated infection. Also, Mercury which rules the structural disorders of epithelial and mucosal lining of urinary tract is occupied in sixth cusp afflicted with Ketu causes recurring infection and inflammation of epithelial and mucosal lining of urinary and genital tract. Sun being lord of eleventh cusp is placed in seventh cusp with sign Aries causes reduced immunity and functional disorder of lymph nodes which secrets various immunoglobulin in body to form antibodies that prevents the infection in body and being it placed in seventh cusp indicates severe and recurring infection and inflammation of genital tract and urinary tract. Also, Sun is under direct aspect of Uranus from ascendant which is known as causative of mysterious diseases that are known to be difficult to diagnose. Also, it is evident that Sun is main source of energy or ruler of dephosphorylation in which ATP molecule releases energy by getting converted into ADP. And as such the native always feels energy less or devoid of stamina to fight with day to day adversaries. Further Mars is placed in tenth house which aspect fifth house causing functional disorders of the genital organs. Jupiter that gives strength to fight with infections is occupied in ninth house with sign Gemini and is under aspect of Rahu gives depleted strength to fight with diseases. Also, Saturn which is known to cause chronic diseases and disorders is occupied in eleventh house aspects fifth house of which Saturn is lord indicating severe and chronic types of infections which normally repeatedly occur and are likely to cause infertility in native. In this chart Neptune occupies second cusp with sign Scorpio and aspect Venus which is lord of ascendant and denotes diseases related to genital organs and as such indicates repeated and severe infectious diseases of genital tract and urinary tract. Specific of this chart is sign Aquarius occupying fifth house which indicates infertility due to structural disorders that are noticed when inflammation of epithelial tissue in urinary tract occurs.

According to KP system also it can be revealed in this chart that, star lord of ascendant Mars which is placed in tenth house aspect the fifth house indicating occurrence of disease related; Mars is also star lord of fifth house. Star lord of sixth house Jupiter which is also sub lord of twelfth house is placed in ninth house and in quadrant with Ketu and Rahu denotes the occurrence of disease related to urinary tract. Sub lord of ascendant is occupied in sixth cusp afflicted with Ketu causes the onset of infections. Sub lord of eighth cusp Rah is placed in twelfth house aspects the sub lord of ascendant and in quadrant with Sub lord of twelfth house Jupiter indicating the chronic nature of the disease. As it was noticed that the onset of infection occurred when Saturn mahadasha was in progress and Jupiter antardasha with Mars antardasha period in November 2002; here Jupiter and Mars are star lord and sub lord of sixth house, respectively.

## Planetary Longitudes and disposition

| Planet | Zodiac | Degrees | Lord Zodiac | Star Lord | Sub Lord |
|---|---|---|---|---|---|
| Sun | Aries | 190:24:57 | Mars | Ketu | Saturn |
| Moon | Libra | 028:21:29 | Venus | Jupiter | Venus |
| Mars | Cancer | 281:41:00 | Moon | Saturn | Moon |
| Mercury | Pisces | 171:10:34 | Jupiter | Mercury | Venus |
| Jupiter | Gemini | 248:22:57 | Mercury | Rahu | Rahu |
| Venus | Taurus | 213:01:23 | Venus | Sun | Saturn |
| Saturn | Leo | 300:05:50 | Sun | Ketu | Ketu |
| Rahu | Virgo | 340:59:16 | Mercury | Moon | Moon |
| Ketu | Pisces | 160:59:16 | Jupiter | Saturn | Sun |
| Uranus. | Libra | 021:17:09 | Venus | Jupiter | Jupiter |
| Neptune. | Scorpio | 054:27:05 | Mars | Mercury | Rahu |

## KP house divisions and Lord of cusps

| Cusp | Zodiac | Lord of Zodiac | Star Lord | Sub Lord |
|---|---|---|---|---|
| 01 | Libra | Venus | Mars | Mercury |
| 02 | Libra | Venus | Jupiter | Moon |
| 03 | Scorpio | Mars | Mercury | Saturn |
| 04 | Sagittarius | Jupiter | Sun | Rahu |
| 05 | Aquarius | Saturn | Mars | Mercury |
| 06 | Pisces | Jupiter | Jupiter | Mars |
| 07 | Aries | Mars | Ketu | Ketu |
| 08 | Aries | Mars | Sun | Rahu |

| Cusp | Zodiac | Lord of Zodiac | Star Lord | Sub Lord |
|------|--------|----------------|-----------|----------|
| 09 | Taurus | Venus | Mars | Saturn |
| 10 | Gemini | Mercury | Jupiter | Moon |
| 11 | Leo | Sun | Ketu | Ketu |
| 12 | Virgo | Mercury | Sun | Jupiter |

Case No. 005/trm

Native born on 05<sup>th</sup> April 1992 at 16:50 hours in Jalgaon with Lat. 021:06 Long. 075:36E

This is case again a Leo ascendant and lord of ascendant placed in eighth house conjoined with Mercury which is lord of second and eleventh house and Venus which is lord of third and tenth cusp. Further Jupiter which imparts strength to fight with infections is placed in ascendant. Fifth house is occupied by Uranus, Neptune, and Rahu and as such afflicting the cusp indicates occurrence of infectious diseases. Lord of seventh cusp Saturn is placed in sixth cusp with own sign Capricorn; this indicates repeated and inflammation and infection of urinary and genital tract. Seventh house is afflicted with Mars being occupied in Aquarius which indicates structural disorders and as such cause's serious infection of mucosal and epithelial lining of internal wall of urinary tract and genital tract. Further Venus which is ruler of functions of genital tract is placed in eighth cusp and in quadrant with Rahu and Ketu causes recurring inflammation of urinary tract. Also Mercury which rules the structure of mucosal layer of urinary and genital tract is occupied in eighth cusp and also in quadrant of Uranus causes the structural disorders of the internal wall of urinary and genital tract. Because of Jupiter placed in ascendant gives some relief from these malefic effects by increasing the immunity and timely responding to the drugs administered.

According to KP system it is further revealed that Sub lord of ascendant Ketu is placed in eleventh house aspect fifth cusp indicating the repeated infection or diseases related with urinary tract. Also, star lord of ascendant Venus is occupied in eighth cusp conjoined with star lord of twelfth cusp and star lord of eighth cusp Mercury indicating severity of disease. The Star lord of sixth house Mars is placed in seventh house causes onset of the disease in the dasha lord of Mars. Also Sub lord of twelfth house Jupiter is placed in ascendant aspects the fifth house and occupant Rahu which is sub lord of eighth house causes the infection and inflammation. As such ascendant, sixth cusp, eighth cusp and twelfth cusp are well connected indicating the infection and inflammation of urinary and genital tract.

The occurrence of infection was first noticed and reported in April 2019 when Mars mahadasha Mars antardasha and pratiantardasha of Jupiter; where Mars is Star lord of sixth house and Jupiter is sub lord of sixth cusp which confirms the KP theory

Planetary longitudes and disposition is tabled as given below.

| Planet | Zodiac | Degrees | Lord zodiac | Star Lord | Sub Lord |
|---|---|---|---|---|---|
| Sun | Scorpio | 146:45:07 | Mars | Mercury | Jupiter |
| Moon | Libra | 068:58:00 | Venus | Rahu | Jupiter |
| Mars | Taurus | 216:39:18 | Venus | Sun | Mercury |
| Mercury | Sagittarius | 135:54:17 | Jupiter | Venus | Sun |
| Jupiter | Cancer | 349:36:07 | Moon | Mercury | Venus |
| Venus | Sagittarius | 126:52:09 | Jupiter | Ketu | Rahu |
| Saturn | Sagittarius | 149:47:00 | Jupiter | Sun | Rahu |
| Rahu | Capricorn | 156:24:42 | Saturn | Sun | Mercury |
| Ketu | Cancer | 336:24:42 | Moon | Saturn | Mercury |
| Uranus | Sagittarius | 134:51:28 | Jupiter | Venus | Venus |
| Neptune | Sagittarius | 139:40:24 | Jupiter | Venus | Rahu |

## KP House Division and Lord of Cusp

| Cusp | Zodiac | Lord of Zodiac | Star Lord | Sub Lord |
|---|---|---|---|---|
| 01 | Leo | Sun | Venus | Saturn |
| 02 | Virgo | Mercury | Moon | Sun |
| 03 | Libra | Venus | Jupiter | Saturn |
| 04 | Scorpio | Mars | Mercury | Mars |
| 05 | Sagittarius | Jupiter | Venus | Mercury |
| 06 | Capricorn | Saturn | Mars | Rahu |
| 07 | Aquarius | Saturn | Jupiter | Saturn |
| 08 | Pisces | Jupiter | Mercury | Moon |
| 09 | Aries | Mars | Venus | Saturn |
| 10 | Taurus | Venus | Mars | Mars |
| 11 | Gemini | Mercury | Jupiter | Mercury |
| 12 | Cancer | Moon | Mercury | Rahu |

Case No. 006/ns
The native born on 03rd May 1995 at 19:10 hours Aurangabad
Lat. 019:48N Long. 075:19E

This is also classic birth chart that gives us an idea how planetary longitudes denote the exact type, cause, and time of onset of disease with intensity and aftereffects. It is Libra ascendant chart and lord of ascendant is placed in sixth cusp with sign Pisces. Venus rules the function of reproductive organs and sixth cusp is cusp that rules diseases and disorders. Rahu is placed in ascendant indicating weak constitution of physiological wellbeing. Jupiter that imparts the strength to fight with diseases and disorders is placed in second cusp with sign Scorpio and is in quincunx with Ketu occupied in seventh house indicating weakness. Fourth cusp is severely afflicted with Uranus conjoined with Neptune in sign Capricorn indicating Pelvic diseases. Saturn lord of fourth and fifth house is placed in fifth house in own sign Aquarius and as we know Saturn rules obstructive and chronic diseases and disorders causes serious and severe Pelvic Inflammation Disease. Further Sun that rules the function of lymph nodes and immunoglobulin's; cause extremely poor immunity and as such recurring infections which are difficult to recover. Sun is placed in seventh house afflicted with Ketu with sign Aries gives structural disorders of mucosal membranes of genital tract and leads to infections. Mercury which is known to rule epithelial and mucosal layers of urinary and genital tract is occupied in eighth cusp with sign Taurus gives dryness of the lining causing growth of fungal and bacterial organisms in urinary and genital tract. Moon which is known to rule functions of secretary glands in human body and hormones is placed in ninth house in quincunx with Uranus and Neptune indicating functional disorders of secretary glands and lymph nodes which secrets immunoglobulin causing hormonal disorders and lowered immunity. Mars which is lord of seventh cusp is placed in tenth house with sign Canceris under aspect of Uranus and Neptune and aspect fifth house indicating severe infection and inflammation of urinary tract, genital tract and leads to pelvic inflammation. Pelvic Inflammation Disease is known to cause blockages of fallopian tubes and obstructs the menstrual periods cause infertility.

According to KP cusp study it reveals that star lord of sixth house Mercury is occupied in eighth cusp and star lord of eighth cusp Moon is placed in ninth cusp in Gemini, a sign owned by Mercury. Also, star lord of twelfth cusp is placed in tenth cusp aspect Saturn which is sub lord of ascendant. Further sub lord of sixth cusp and twelfth cusp Jupiter is occupied in second house aspect Mars which is star lord of twelfth cusp. Sun which is sub lord of eighth cusp is placed in seventh house afflicted with Ketu. This indicates the occurrence of the disease but not the severity or intensity of the disease which means the infection will occur but may not become chronic and severe. The occurrence of disease if noticed it clarifies that in moth of March the first infection was reported to doctors in moth of March 2017 when mahadasha and antardasha of Jupiter was in progress where Jupiter is sub lord of sixth cusp and pratiantardasha of Mercury which is star lord of sixth cusp. The native reported was recovered when Jupiter antardasha was over that is in January 2019.

Planetary longitudes and disposition are tabled herewith

| Planet | zodiac | Degrees | Lord of zodiac | Star lord | Sub lord |
|---|---|---|---|---|---|
| Sun | Aries | 198:52:10 | Mars | Venus | Rahu |
| Moon | Gemini | 240:44:40 | Mercury | Mars | Mercury |
| Mars | Cancer | 297:15:49 | Moon | Mercury | Jupiter |
| Mercury | Taurus | 217:41:32 | Venus | Sun | Ketu |
| Jupiter | Scorpio | 050:02:54 | Mars | Mercury | Venus |
| Venus | Pisces | 169:58:46 | Jupiter | Mercury | Venus |
| Saturn | Aquarius | 147:47:44 | Saturn | Jupiter | Venus |
| Rahu | Libra | 011:28:43 | Venus | Rahu | Saturn |
| Ketu | Aries | 191:28:43 | Mars | Ketu | Mercury |
| Uranus | Capricorn | 096:40:44 | Saturn | Sun | Mercury |
| Neptune | Capricorn | 091:44:50 | Saturn | Sun | Jupiter |

## KP House divisions and lords of cusp

| Cusp | Zodiac | Lord of zodiac | Star Lord | Sub Lord |
|---|---|---|---|---|
| 01 | Libra | Venus | Jupiter | Saturn |
| 02 | Scorpio | Mars | Mercury | Moon |
| 03 | Sagittarius | Jupiter | Venus | Saturn |
| 04 | Capricorn | Saturn | Mars | Rahu |

| Cusp | Zodiac | Lord of zodiac | Star Lord | Sub Lord |
|------|--------|----------------|-----------|----------|
| 05 | Aquarius | Saturn | Jupiter | Venus |
| 06 | Pisces | Jupiter | Mercury | Jupiter |
| 07 | Aries | Mars | Venus | Saturn |
| 08 | Taurus | Venus | Moon | Sun |
| 09 | Gemini | Mercury | Jupiter | Saturn |
| 10 | Cancer | Moon | Mercury | Rahu |
| 11 | Leo | Sun | Sun | Venus |
| 12 | Virgo | Mercury | Mars | Jupiter |

Case No. 007/mrk

Native born on 13th May 1987 at 01:00 hours in Nanded city

Lat. 019:09 N Long. 077:18E

This chart is typical of Capricorn ascendant and is classic to study the combination of structural as well as functional disorders of urinary and genital tract that becomes chronic leading to serious surgical procedures required to remove uterus.

The lord of ascendant Saturn is placed in eleventh cusp and aspect fifth house occupied by Mercury which rules the epithelial and mucosal layers of urinary tract indicating severe and chronic infection. Jupiter that protects the body by imparting strength to fight with infections is placed in third cusp afflicted with Rahu and under aspect of Ketu. This naturally reduces the immunity causing infection and inflammation. Sun which is lord of eighth cusp is occupied in fourth cusp with sign Aries and conjoined with lord of fifth house; this indicates the severe inflammation of urinary tract leading to structural disorder of the mucosal wall. Fifth house is occupied by Mercury which is lord of sixth cusp denotes severe infection of urinary and genital tract. Also, lord of fourth cusp Mars is placed in sixth cusp indicating recurring and difficult to diagnose disorders of urinary tract which may sometimes spread to bladder and kidneys. Also, Mars is under aspect of Uranus and Neptune occupied in twelfth house indicates frequent dysfunctional bleeding. The lord of seventh house Moon is placed in tenth house under aspect of Sun which is lord of eighth cusp and in quincunx with Rahu occupied in third cusp. It is noticeable here that lord of ascendant Saturn is placed in eleventh cusp with sign Scorpio and aspect fifth house

and Mercury indicating obstructive structural disorder of genital tract. According to KP cusp analysis also it is clear here to note that star lord of ascendant is placed in sixth cusp and is in quadrant with Jupiter which is star lord of sixth cusp. Further star lord of eighth cusp Sun which is also star lord of twelfth cusp is placed in fourth cusp with sign Aries indicates occurrence of the severe infection of epithelial and mucosal lining of urinary and genital tract; Sun is also sub lord of sixth house. Also sub lord of ascendant Saturn is occupied in eleventh cusp and aspect sub lord of eighth cusp Mercury and in quincunx with Mars, sub lord of twelfth house; this clarifies the recurring and chronic type of structural disorders of lining of urinary tract and genital tract. The occurrence of the infection first noticed in March 2016; when mahadasha Saturn was in progress. And antardasha of Sun was concluding with last pratiantardasha of Jupiter. Here Jupiter is star lord of sixth house and Sun is sub lord of sixth house. When we study the birth chart microscopically we find that though the infection was actually reported in March 2016 must have occurred much earlier may be in the month of May 2000 as it appears that in Jupiter mahadasha and antardasha of Sun some infection would have occurred but due to strength of Jupiter during the period was easily controlled. This time the native was required to shift to hospital and get the treatment.

## Planetary longitudes and disposition

| Planet | Zodiac | Degrees | Lord Zodiac | Star Lord | Sub Lord |
|---|---|---|---|---|---|
| Sun | Aries | 147:51:45 | Mars | Sun | Moon |
| Moon | Libra | 288:13:12 | Venus | Rahu | Moon |
| Mars | Gemini | 150:53:51 | Mercury | Mars | Mercury |
| Mercury | Taurus | 124:19:42 | Venus | Sun | Saturn |
| Jupiter | Pisces | 083:06:41 | Jupiter | Mercury | Moon |
| Venus | Aries | 120:39:03 | Mars | Ketu | Ketu |
| Saturn | Scorpio | 326:05:41 | Mars | Mercury | Rahu |
| Rahu | Pisces | 075:50:06 | Jupiter | Saturn | Jupiter |
| Ketu | Virgo | 255:50:06 | Mercury | Moon | Saturn |
| Uranus | Sagitta. | 332:21:16 | Jupiter | Ketu | Venus |
| Neptune | Sagitta. | 344:02:35 | Jupiter | Venus | Venus |

KP Divisions and Lords of Cusp

| Cusp | Zodiacs | Lord of Zodiac | Star Lord | Sub Lord |
|---|---|---|---|---|
| 01 | Capricorn | Saturn | Mars | Saturn |
| 02 | Pisces | Jupiter | Saturn | Mercury |
| 03 | Aries | Mars | Ketu | Saturn |
| 04 | Taurus | Venus | Sun | Venus |
| 05 | Gemini | Mercury | Mars | Venus |
| 06 | Gemini | Mercury | Jupiter | Sun |
| 07 | Cancer | Moon | Mercury | Saturn |
| 08 | Virgo | Mercury | Sun | Mercury |
| 09 | Libra | Venus | Rahu | Jupiter |
| 10 | Scorpio | Mars | Saturn | Venus |
| 11 | Sagittarius | Jupiter | Ketu | Sun |
| 12 | Sagittarius | Jupiter | Sun | Mars |

Planetary disposition in cases of uterine disease Uterine problems as we have discussed earlier are mainly functional abnormalities and occur when hormonal imbalance is noticed, or menstrual irregularities observed and also when some typical psychological symptoms are noticed. We have discussed few cases of uterine problems which occur normally in the range of age group of 18 to 35.

Case No. 008/spb
Native birth date is 13th July 1975 at 11:33 hrs in Udgir
Lat. 018:24 N Long. 077:06 E

This is Virgo ascendant chart and lord of ascendant placed in tenth cusp afflicted with Saturn and Sun with sign Gemini. Uranus occupied in second house with sign Libra which aspect Mars placed in eighth house which is lord of third and eighth cusp. Neptune conjoined with Rahu occupied in third cusp with sign Scorpio aspect ninth house. Jupiter lord of fourth and seventh house is occupied in seventh house with own sign Pisces. Moon lord of eleventh cusp is placed in twelfth house with sign Leo and conjoined with Venus which is lord of ninth and second house. In this chart fifth house which in Time Personified natural chart rules the genital organs and urinary tract is occupied by Capricorn and under quincunx with Saturn and lord of twelfth house Sun indicating infertility due to structural disorders. Mars placed in eighth cusp denotes functional disorders and as such causes Amenorrhea which means absence of menstruation periods consecutively for more than six months. Moon placed in twelfth house indicates hormonal disorders due to growth of adhesions developed in uterus as fifth house is under quincunx with Saturn. Also as lord twelfth house occupied in tenth house conjoined with lord of fifth house causes obstructive growth of lesions and cysts in ovaries. Giving rise to poor or no secretion of hormones leading to poor or no ovulation as confirmed after the specific tests conducted by doctors indicating disturbed FSH and prolactin levels. Also, tests conducted for ovarian cysts indicated by Antimulerian Hormone tests.

This further was confirmed by various USG tests and medicated for long period failure to which got operated for removal of one side entire ovary. Because of Saturn occupied conjoined with Sun the recurring growth of poly cystic ovarian disorders led to ultimately infertility.

After almost ten years again when severe abdominal pain was reported and got tested for USG it was found that this time some adhesions were found developed in uterus; this caused hysterectomy. Few points which must be taken into account are the aspect or any type of relation of fifth cusp with Saturn certainly gives obstructive type of structural disorders, also when lord of twelfth house conjoins with lord of fifth cusp produces repeated growth of cysts in ovaries causing functional disorders of ovaries; and thirdly because Moon which rules the secretary function of hormones and causes ovulation is placed in twelfth house and also under aspect of Saturn from tenth cusp causes severe various functional complications that lead to permanent infertility. Interesting here is to note further that Mars occupied in eighth house also causes dysfunctional bleeding and growth of polycystic ovarian disorder. All these points were first noted and native was asked to take help of skilled gynaecologist but went in vein as it became recurring problem till the hysterectomy was carried out.

The native first visited when was for when her marriage will take place but after the birth chart was studied asked to contact doctor urgently as the Amenorrhea was unnoticed for long time. And birth chart revealed the further complications. This occurred in April 1995 when Moon mahadasha and Ketuantardasha was progressing. The native got recovered after treatment and got married in 2000 Mars1 March and within short period of couple of years again the problem repeatedly occurred, indicating severe abdominal pain and amenorrhea. This time doctor advised to remove uterus as severe adhesion and abnormal growth is observed in USG. The second time native reported on 10th May 2015 when she was advised by doctors to prepare for hysterectomy and as such was operated for hysterectomy on 28th December 2015when Rahu mahadasha and Ketu antardasha was in progress and Ketu pratiantardasha was just started. In this case Rahu is star lord of sixth cusp and Ketu is sub lord of sixth cusp. According to KP system also it reveals that star lord of ascendant Moon is occupied in twelfth cusp with star lord of twelfth cusp Venus and aspect sixth house as well as under aspect of lord of sixth house. Also star sixth cusp is occupied in third cusp aspect Star lord of twelfth cusp conjoined with Moon; Venus is also star lord of eighth cusp. Further sub lord of ascendant Jupiter is occupied in seventh cusp aspect ascendant, also sub lord of sixth cusp Ketu is placed in ninth house in quadrant with Venus which is sub lord of eighth and twelfth cusp and thus well connecting ascendant, sixth cusp, eighth cusp and twelfth cusp. This indicates the hospitalization followed by surgical procedure.

## Planetary longitudes and disposition

| Planet | Zodiac | Degrees | Lord of Zodiac | Star Lord | Sub Lord |
|---|---|---|---|---|---|
| Sun | Gemini | 296:43:43 | Mercury | Jupiter | Venus |
| Moon | Leo | 352:25:21 | Sun | Venus | Saturn |
| Mars | Aries | 224:59:03 | Mars | Venus | Venus |
| Mercury | Gemini | 277:48:10 | Mercury | Rahu | Rahu |
| Jupiter | Pisces | 209:29:58 | Jupiter | Mercury | Saturn |
| Venus | Leo | 339:08:32 | Sun | Ketu | Jupiter |
| Saturn | Gemini | 298:40:29 | Mercury | Jupiter | Venus |
| Rahu | Scorpio | 064:50:17 | Mars | Saturn | Saturn |
| Ketu | Taurus | 244:50:17 | Venus | Sun | Saturn |
| Uranus | Libra | 034:51:17 | Venus | Mars | Venus |
| Neptune | Scorpio | 075:53:38 | Mars | Saturn | Jupiter |

## KP House Divisions and Lords of Cusp

| Cusp | Zodiac | Lord of Zodiac | Star Lord | Sub Lord |
|------|--------|----------------|-----------|----------|
| 01 | Virgo | Mercury | Moon | Jupiter |
| 02 | Libra | Venus | Rahu | Mercury |
| 03 | Scorpio | Mars | Saturn | Rahu |
| 04 | Sagittarius | Jupiter | Venus | Venus |
| 05 | Capricorn | Saturn | Moon | Jupiter |
| 06 | Aquarius | Saturn | Rahu | Ketu |
| 07 | Pisces | Jupiter | Saturn | Rahu |
| 08 | Aries | Mars | Venus | Venus |
| 09 | Taurus | Venus | Moon | Jupiter |
| 10 | Gemini | Mercury | Rahu | Mercury |
| 11 | Cancer | Moon | Saturn | Rahu |
| 12 | Leo | Sun | Venus | Venus |

## Case 009/mrd

Native born on 07th December 1985 at 09:30 hrs in Aurangabad with Lat. 019:48 N Long. 075:19 E

This chart is typical and denotes the functional and structural abnormalities those were observed during the progress of disorders. So also, it is important to notice the behavioural changes observed in native during the progress of the disorders. In this chart Showing Sagittarius falls in ascendant occupied with Neptune indicates the dissociative personality disorder in native, that is cranky and abnormal behavior after the hormonal disorders started appearing. The lord of ascendant Jupiter is placed in second cusp with sign Capricorn denotes the lack of strength to fight with diseases and physical disorders and as it is placed under aspect of Saturn causes growth of sub mucosal fibroids in uterus. Further Moon which rules the hormonal secretions is lord of eighth cusp placed in tenth cusp in quincunx with Rahu occupied in fifth cusp indicating functional disorders of ovarian function leading to hormonal disorders. Fifth house occupied by Rahu is also under aspect of Mars from eleventh cusp denotes structural disorders as growth of adhesions in uterus and cysts in ovaries. Also, Mars is lord of fifth house and is afflicted with Ketu indicating inflammation of uterine wall and Pelvic inflammation disease. Lord of sixth cusp Venus is placed in twelfth cusp severely afflicted with Saturn and Uranus indicates chronic and obstructive disorders of uterus and causes growth of fibroids in uterus. Also, lord of seventh house Mercury is occupied in twelfth cusp afflicted with Saturn and Uranus indicates abnormalities associated with mucosal and epithelial lining of uterine wall and cervix. This causes growth of adhesions and fibroids in uterus. It can also be noticed that lord of ninth cusp Sun which imparts the immunity and normally prevents the abnormal growth of cells anywhere in body and also gives energy to overcome the abnormalities is placed in twelfth cusp afflicted with Saturn and Uranus causes abnormal structural changes in uterine wall and as such growth of adhesions and fibroids take place. It is noteworthy here that Mars is lord of fifth cusp as well as lord of twelfth cusp occupied in eleventh cusp clearly indicates the serious anomalies associated with uterus to occur. It is interesting to note that first the abnormalities were noticed in April 1997 when native approached doctor for severe abdominal pain and doctor found fibroid growth in ovaries which was removed by surgery. This happened in mahadasha of Mars with antardasha of Ketu and pratiantardasha of also Ketu was just started. Where Mars and Ketu are star lord and sub lord of sixth house. The native led a normal life till June 2017 when again sudden dysfunctional bleeding occurred and native was admitted to hospital and when diagnosed was found to have developed several adhesions in uterine wall which was again required to be surgically removed. This was occurred again in mahadasha Rahu was in progress and antardasha of Mars and pratiantardasha of Ketu. Surprisingly when native was under treatment for infertility disorder for several years never it was noticed any cause of infertility except absence of one ovary which was removed much earlier.

According to KP system also it reveals that star lord of ascendant Sun is occupied in twelfth cusp afflicted with Saturn and Uranus. Also, star lord of sixth cusp Mars is occupied in eleventh house afflicted with star lord of eighth and twelfth cusp Ketu. Further the sub lord of ascendant is placed in tenth house in quincunx with Rahu. sub lord of eighth cusp and twelfth cusp is Venus placed in twelfth cusp with star lord of ascendant indicates the complicated uterine disorders that creates infertility and malfunctioning of ovaries. It is especially important to note here that as fifth house plays a vital role in uterine functions twelfth house is equally important to be considered to find out the malefic effects. As in this case lord of fifth house and lord of eighth house Mars is afflicted.

## Planetary longitudes and disposition

| Planet | Zodiac | Degrees | Lord of Zodiac | Star Lord | Sub Lord |
| --- | --- | --- | --- | --- | --- |
| Sun | Scorpio | 351:19:51 | Mars | Mercury | Venus |
| Moon | Virgo | 284:11:21 | Mercury | Moon | Jupiter |
| Mars | Libra | 301:37:33 | Venus | Mars | Mercury |
| Mercury | Scorpio | 335:15:47 | Mars | Saturn | Saturn |
| Jupiter | Capricorn | 049:43:26 | Saturn | Moon | Ketu |
| Venus | Scorpio | 340:54:07 | Mars | Saturn | Sun |
| Saturn | Scorpio | 338:43:29 | Mars | Saturn | Venus |
| Rahu | Aries | 133:28:48 | Mars | Venus | Venus |
| Ketu | Libra | 313:28:48 | Venus | Rahu | Mercury |
| Uranus | Scorpio | 354:20:49 | Mars | Merc | Rahu |
| Neptune | Sagittarius | 008:59:51 | Jupiter | Ketu | Jupiter |

## KP House Divisions and Lords of Cusp

| Cusp | Zodiac | Lord of Zodiac | Star Lord | Sub Lord |
| --- | --- | --- | --- | --- |
| 01 | Sagittarius | Jupiter | Sun | Moon |
| 02 | Aquarius | Saturn | Mars | Ketu |
| 03 | Pisces | Jupiter | Saturn | Ketu |
| 04 | Aries | Mars | Ketu | Saturn |
| 05 | Taurus | Venus | Sun | Ketu |
| 06 | Gemini | Mercury | Mars | Ketu |
| 07 | Gemini | Mercury | Jupiter | Venus |
| 08 | Leo | Sun | Ketu | Venus |
| 09 | Leo | Sun | Ketu | Venus |
| 10 | Libra | Venus | Rahu | Jupiter |
| 11 | Scorpio | Mars | Saturn | Mercury |
| 12 | Sagittarius | Jupiter | Ketu | Venus |

Case No. 010/aas
Birth date 18<sup>th</sup> July 1983 at 06:05 hours in Sholapur with
Lat. 017:42 N Long. 075:55 E

This chart is typical of Cancer ascendant and in this case, Mars is specific significator of health which in this chart is placed in twelfth cup denoting specific structural disorders of fifth house as it is lord of fifth and tenth house. The lord of ascendant is occupied in fourth cusp afflicted with lord pf eighth and seventh cusp Saturn indicating chronic obstructive diseases of uterus and related organs and Moon being afflicted denotes the functional disorders like hormonal imbalance. Moon being placed in fourth cusp also indicates diminished Luteinizing Hormone and Follicle Stimulating Hormone giving temporary infertility. As in this case fifth house is hemmed in between Saturn in fourth cusp and Neptune causes serious uterine disorders especially structural disorders and as such the native is normally found to have infected with HPV (Human Papilloma Virus) which accelerates the mutation chain in tissue of uterine wall leading to cancerous growth. Further lord of sixth cup Jupiter is placed in fifth house afflicted with Ketu and Uranus. Sun, lord of second house is placed in ascendant and is under aspect of Saturn causes growth of abnormal cells giving rise to tumors. Sun is conjoined with Mercury which is lord of twelfth house also causes severe inflammation of mucosal membrane of uterus. According to KP divisions if we study it is noticed that star lord of ascendant Jupiter is occupied in fifth cusp afflicted with star lord of sixth cusp Ketu indicating uterine diseases. Also, star lord of eighth cusp Mars is placed in twelfth house; Mars is also star lord of twelfth cusp. Further sub lord of ascendant Rahu is occupied in eleventh cusp aspect fifth house is in quadrant with Venus sub lord of sixth cusp placed in second house and aspect Ketu star lord of sixth house and sub lord of twelfth cusp; also Rahu aspect Jupiter which is sub lord of eighth cusp indicating serious inflammatory diseases of uterus. In this case first occurrence of uterine inflammation was noticed in December 2000 when mahadasha of Jupiter was in progress Native with antardasha of Ketu and pratiantardasha of Venus. This time surgical procedure to remove the fibroid was successful and discharged from hospital as totally recovered. There after again the cancerous growth was noticed when dysfunctional bleeding started on 8<sup>th</sup> September 2019. This time mahadasha of Saturn antardasha of Venus was in progress and pratiantardasha of Ketu was started.

In this case Venus is sub lord of sixth cusp and Ketu is star lord of sixth cusp. Native remained unmarried till date for physical debility and psychological distress.

## Planetary Longitudes and disposition case no 010/aas

| Planet | Zodiac | Degrees | Lord of Zodiac | Star Lord | Sub Lord |
|---|---|---|---|---|---|
| Sun | Cancer | 001:13:45 | Moon | Jupiter | Mars |
| Moon | Gemini | 342:23:53 | Venus | Rahu | Saturn |
| Mars | Gemini | 348:54:48 | Mercury | Rahu | Moon |
| Mercury | Cancer | 010:43:20 | Moon | Saturn | Sun |
| Jupiter | Scorpio | 127:38:18 | Mars | Saturn | Ketu |
| Venus | Leo | 101:06:44 | Sun | Ketu | Saturn |
| Saturn | Libra | 094:19:25 | Venus | Mars | Venus |
| Rahu | Taurus | 329:45:04 | Venus | Mars | Saturn |
| Ketu | Scorpio | 149:45:04 | Mars | Mercury | Saturn |
| Uranus | Scorpio | 131:45:17 | Mars | Saturn | Moon |
| Neptune | Sagittarius. | 153:30:28 | Jupiter | Ketu | Sun |

## KP House Division and Lords of cusp

| Cusp | Zodiac | Lord of Zodiac | Star Lord | Sub Lord |
|---|---|---|---|---|
| 01 | Cancer | Moon | Jupiter | Rahu |
| 02 | Cancer | Moon | Mercury | Jupiter |
| 03 | Leo | Sun | Venus | Ketu |
| 04 | Virgo | Mercury | Mars | Saturn |
| 05 | Scorpio | Mars | Jupiter | Mars |
| 06 | Sagittarius | Jupiter | Ketu | Venus |
| 07 | Capricorn | Saturn | Sun | Jupiter |
| 08 | Capricorn | Saturn | Mars | Jupiter |
| 09 | Aquarius | Saturn | Jupiter | Ketu |
| 10 | Pisces | Jupiter | Mercury | Saturn |
| 11 | Taurus | Venus | Sun | Rahu |
| 12 | Gemini | Mercury | Mars | Ketu |

Case No. 011/rrn
Native born on 30<sup>th</sup> January 1981 at 15:21 hours in Mumbai with
Lat. 018:57 N Long. 072:49 E

In this case with Gemini ascendant and lord of ascendant Mercury occupied in ninth cusp afflicted with Mars which is lord of sixth cusp with sign Aquarius denotes the weak constitution of the native prone for infectious diseases. This Mercury is also in quadrant with Uranus occupied in sixth house indicating mysterious disorders related to wall of Uterus. Moon which is lord of second house Cancer is placed afflicted with Uranus in sixth house indicates functional disorders specifically related with hormones and certain steroids. Further Sun, lord of third house is occupied in eighth cusp conjoined with Venus which is lord of fifth house and twelfth cusp with sign Capricorn clearly indicates the reduced physical strength to fight against diseases. This also indicates aggressive nature that leads to repetitive imbalance in hormones and blood pressure. Fourth house is occupied by Jupiter lord of seventh house afflicted with Saturn which is lord of eighth house in sign Virgo indicates abnormal growth of cells in wall of uterus that leads to cancer in later stage. Thus, fifth house is found hemmed in between Saturn in fourth cusp and Uranus in sixth cusp denotes serious uterine structural disorders that also lead to functional disorders. Also, seventh house is occupied by Neptune indicates obstructive growth in reproductive organs. it is also important to note here is that Jupiter placed in forth house in sign Virgo is in quincunx with Mercury placed in ninth house which is lord of fourth house causes growth of cancerous cells in uterine wall. Further it is also important to note that lord of twelfth cusp Venus is placed in eighth cusp indicating the serious disorders related to uterus as Venus is also lord of fifth house.

According to KP system also we find star lord of ascendant Mars is occupied in ninth cusp; star lord of sixth cusp Saturn which is also sub lord of sixth and twelfth cusp is placed in fourth cusp in quincunx with Mars. Further star lord of eighth cusp Sun is occupied in eighth house under aspect from Rahu which is sub lord of eighth cusp, Sun is also sub lord of ascendant and indicates serious difficult to recover problems associated with reproductive organs. The onset of the disease was reported in November 2010 when Mahadasha of Ketu with antardasha of Saturn was in progress with Saturn pratiantardasha just started, where Saturn is star lord and sub lord of sixth cusp.

## Planetary Longitudes and disposition

| Planets | Zodiac | Degrees | Lord of Zodiac | Star Lord | Sub Lord |
|---------|--------|---------|----------------|-----------|----------|
| Sun | Capricorn | 226:50:23 | Saturn | Moon | Saturn |
| Moon | Scorpio | 161:16:35 | Mars | Saturn | Moon |
| Mars | Aquarius | 240:26:45 | Saturn | Mars | Mercury |
| Mercury | Aquarius | 244:48:09 | Saturn | Mars | Venus |
| Jupiter | Virgo | 106:04:08 | Mercury | Moon | Saturn |
| Venus | Capricorn | 210:20:49 | Saturn | Sun | Rahu |
| Saturn | Virgo | 106:04:08 | Mercury | Moon | Saturn |
| Rahu | Cancer | 047:22:09 | Moon | Mercury | Mercury |
| Ketu | Capricorn | 227:22:09 | Saturn | Moon | Saturn |
| Uranus | Scorpio | 156:00:50 | Mars | Saturn | Mercury |
| Neptune | Sagittarius | 180:25:57 | Jupiter | Ketu | Ketu |

## KP House divisions and Lords of Cusp

| Cusp | Zodiac | Lord of Zodiac | Star Lord | Sub Lord |
|------|--------|----------------|-----------|----------|
| 01 | Gemini | Mercury | Mars | Sun |
| 02 | Gemini | Mercury | Jupiter | Moon |
| 03 | Cancer | Moon | Mercury | Rahu |
| 04 | Leo | Sun | Venus | Mercury |
| 05 | Virgo | Mercury | Mars | Saturn |
| 06 | Scorpio | Mars | Saturn | Saturn |
| 07 | Sagittarius | Jupiter | Ketu | Mars |
| 08 | Sagittarius | Jupiter | Sun | Rahu |
| 09 | Capricorn | Saturn | Mars | Rahu |
| 10 | Aquarius | Saturn | Jupiter | Mercury |
| 11 | Pisces | Jupiter | Mercury | Saturn |
| 12 | Taurus | Venus | Sun | Saturn |

Case No. 012/ssj

Native born on 23rd February 1978 at 19:30 hours in Mumbai/ Mulund with Lat 019:10 N Long 072:57 E

A classical case describing the entire sequence till the Hysterectomy that gives confirmation of the effect of Birth chart exerted on the native. Leo ascendant chart shows lord of ascendant placed in seventh house in sign Aquarius con joined with Mercury which is lord of eleventh cusp and second cusp and Venus, lord of tenth and third cusp; Sun is under direct aspect of Saturn from first house, where Saturn is lord of sixth house and seventh house. This indicates chronic obstructive and irrecoverable diseases associated with uterus. Also Moon which is lord of twelfth house is occupied in ascendant indicates hormonal and Lymph node related disorders, also as Moon is afflicted with Saturn causes severe functional disorders of endocrine glands and other immunity functions that lead to depletion in cancer antigens in body causing uncontrolled growth of cells anywhere in body. Mars lord of fourth house and ninth house Mars is placed in eleventh house conjoined with Jupiter which is lord of fifth and eighth house and aspect fifth house indicates growth of adhesions in uterine tissues. Lord of fifth cusp and eighth cusp Jupiter aspect fifth cusp and Rahu is placed in quincunx with fifth house denotes abnormal cells growth in uterus which further causes Hysterectomy. In this chart lord of fifth and eighth cusp Jupiter aspect fifth house causing the growth of unwanted cells in tissue of uterine wall. Further seventh house that rules the genital disorders is directly under aspect of Saturn also gives diseases related to reproductive system. When in June2008 the native asked to first visit doctors and then decide regarding the expected pregnancy and remedy for infertility was suffering from unnoticed dysfunctional bleeding. Doctors after thorough examination and respective tests concluded the uterus has developed cancerous growth in wall and surrounding tissues and native was advised hysterectomy and permanent infertility. According to KP system star lord of ascendant Venus is occupied in seventh house conjoined with Sun which is lord of ascendant and Mercury which is star lord of eighth house and star lord of twelfth house. Also, star lord of sixth cusp is occupied in eleventh house aspect Mercury and Venus in seventh house. Further sub lord of ascendant Saturn is occupied in ascendant is conjoined with sub lord of eighth cusp Moon and aspect seventh house. Sub lord of sixth house Mars which is also sub lord of twelfth cusp is placed in eleventh house. As such ascendant, sixth cusp, eighth cusp and twelfth cusp are well connected causing growth of cancer, hospitalization and hysterectomy. The occurrence of this was noticed in June 2008 when mahadasha of Mars, antardasha of Mars and pratiantardasha of Mars was in progress but apparently it may coincide in actual the growth must have started long back which was not on record even irregular menstruation cycles or dysfunctional bleeding or pain in abdomen was totally went unnoticed.

Planetary longitudes and disposition are tabled as under.

| Planets | Zodiac | Degrees | Lord of Zodiac | Star Lord | Sub Lord |
|---|---|---|---|---|---|
| Sun | Aquarius | 191:02:52 | Saturn | Rahu | Saturn |
| Moon | Leo | 017:08:27 | Sun | Venus | Moon |
| Mars | Gemini | 329:01:00 | Mercury | Jupiter | Sun |
| Mercury | Aquarius | 188:05:22 | Saturn | Rahu | Rahu |
| Jupiter | Gemini | 302:32:20 | Mercury | Mars | Ketu |
| Venus | Aquarius | 198:51:05 | Saturn | Rahu | Moon |
| Saturn | Leo | 002:58:51 | Sun | Ketu | Venus |
| Rahu | Virgo | 044:09:49 | Mercury | Moon | Jupiter |
| Ketu | Pisces | 224:09:49 | Jupiter | Saturn | Rahu |
| Uranus | Libra | 082:50:54 | Venus | Jupiter | Saturn |

## KP House Divisions and Lord of Cusp

| Cusp | Zodiac | Lord of Zodiac | Star Lord | Sub Lord |
|---|---|---|---|---|
| 01 | Leo | Sun | Venus | Saturn |
| 02 | Virgo | Mercury | Moon | Venus |
| 03 | Libra | Venus | Jupiter | Saturn |
| 04 | Scorpio | Mars | Mercury | Mars |
| 05 | Sagittarius | Jupiter | Venus | Saturn |
| 06 | Capricorn | Saturn | Mars | Mars |
| 07 | Aquarius | Saturn | Jupiter | Saturn |
| 08 | Pisces | Jupiter | Mercury | Moon |
| 09 | Aries | Mars | Venus | Saturn |
| 10 | Taurus | Venus | Mars | Mars |
| 11 | Gemini | Mercury | Jupiter | Saturn |
| 12 | Cancer | Moon | Mercury | Mars |

Case No. 013/rak
Date of Birth 31st August 1984 at 04:42 hours in Pune with
Lat. 018:36 N Long. 073:48 E

In this Cancer ascendant chart lord of ascendant Moon is occupied in fourth
cusp afflicted with Saturn which is lord of seventh and eighth cusp and as
such at first instance indicates that the hormone secretary system and ovaries
are having functional disorders. Further Sun which is lord of second house is

placed in own sign Leo in second cusp afflicted with Mercury which is lord of eighth cusp gives constant low energy levels causing diseases to occur. Also, fifth house is occupied by Mars which is lord of tenth and fifth house in own sign Scorpio afflicted with malefic like Ketu and Uranus that indicates mysterious severe infection and inflammation. Further sixth house is occupied by Jupiter lord of ninth and sixth house afflicted with Neptune that repeatedly causes infectious growth of fungus or bacteria. This also observed from the chart that fifth cusp is hemmed in between Saturn in fourth cusp and Neptune in sixth cusp certain to cause severe infection of PID type (Pelvic Inflammation Disease) that is also likely to cause structural disorders in cervix and uterus. It is also observed that Rahu occupied in eleventh house in sign Taurus aspect fifth house giving cause to infections and inflammations. In this chart it is also observed that Saturn placed in fourth cusp causes painful menstruation and severe back pain.

According to KP system also it can be understood that the Pelvic Inflammation Disease is certain to occur. As star lord of ascendant Mercury is placed with Sun and Mercury is also lord of twelfth cusp. Star lord of sixth cusp Venus is placed in third house in Virgo and star lord of eighth cusp Rahu is occupied in eleventh cusp is in quincunx with Jupiter placed in sixth house which is star lord of twelfth house; this clearly indicates that during the period of Dasha lord of sixth house infection will occur. Further it is also evident that Sub lord of ascendant Venus is placed in quadrant with Jupiter which is sub lord of twelfth house and aspect Sun which is sub lord of eighth cusp; this confirms the occurrence of severe infection in uterus or ovaries. As observed it was noticed that the native suffered severe infection in abdomen and when approached doctor it was confirmed that it was Pelvic Inflammation Disease which caused hospitalization, this happened in month of April 2003 when Jupiter mahadasha was in progress with onset of antardasha and pratiantardasha of Venus. Here Jupiter is sub lord of sixth house and Venus is star lord of sixth cusp.

Planetary longitudes and disposition are given herewith as under.

| Planet | Zodiac | Degrees | Lord of zodiac | Star Lord | Sub Lord |
|---|---|---|---|---|---|
| Sun | Leo | 044:05:44 | Sun | Venus | Venus |
| Moon | Libra | 102:16:12 | Venus | Rahu | Saturn |

| Planet | Zodiac | Degrees | Lord of zodiac | Star Lord | Sub Lord |
|---|---|---|---|---|---|
| Mars | Scorpio | 133:41:39 | Mars | Saturn | Rahu |
| Mercury | Leo | 039:44:41 | Sun | Ketu | Saturn |
| Jupiter | Sagittarius | 159:29:17 | Jupiter | Ketu | Saturn |
| Venus | Virgo | 064:49:51 | Mercury | Sun | Saturn |
| Saturn | Libra | 107:55:07 | Venus | Rahu | Sun |
| Rahu | Taurus | 308:01:37 | Venus | Sun | Venus |
| Ketu | Scorpio | 128:01:37 | Mars | Ketu | Saturn |
| Uranus | Scorpio | 135:57:51 | Mars | Saturn | Jupiter |
| Neptune | Sagittarius | 155:02:32 | Jupiter | Ketu | Mars |

## KP House Divisions and Lords of Cusp

| Cusp | Zodiac | Lord of Zodiac | Star Lord | Sub Lord |
|---|---|---|---|---|
| 01 | Cancer | Moon | Mercury | Venus |
| 02 | Leo | Sun | Venus | Mars |
| 03 | Virgo | Mercury | Moon | Mercury |
| 04 | Libra | Venus | Jupiter | Jupiter |
| 05 | Scorpio | Mars | Mercury | Venus |
| 06 | Sagittarius | Jupiter | Venus | Jupiter |
| 07 | Capricorn | Saturn | Moon | Venus |
| 08 | Aquarius | Saturn | Rahu | Sun |
| 09 | Pisces | Jupiter | Mercury | Mercury |
| 10 | Aries | Mars | Venus | Rahu |
| 11 | Taurus | Venus | Moon | Venus |
| 12 | Gemini | Mercury | Jupiter | Jupiter |

Case No. 014/aam
Native born on 27th October 1985 at 00:15 hrs in Mumbai with
Lat. 019:03 N Long. 072:52 E

This is Cancer ascendant chart with lord of ascendant placed in ninth cusp
with sign Pisces in quincunx with Ketu occupied in fourth cusp. Also, Sun
lord of second cusp is occupied I n fourth house afflicted with Ketu and lord of
twelfth cusp Mercury indicating functional disorders of mucosal or epithelial
lining anywhere in body and reduces immunity. Further lord of tenth and
fifth cusp Mars is occupied in third house with sign Virgo and conjoined with

Venus which is lord of fourth and eleventh house. Saturn which is lord of eighth cusp and seventh cusp is occupied in fifth cusp afflicted with Uranus; this indicates obstructive, inflammatory and mysterious diseases related to uterus. Neptune is occupied in sixth house with sign Sagittarius; lord of sixth house and ninth cusp is occupied in seventh house which indicates inflammatory diseases associated with uterus. It is evident here that fifth house is hemmed in between Ketu in fourth house and Neptune in sixth house causes functional disorders related to uterus or ovaries. Fifth house is also in quincunx with Rahu placed in tenth cusp and lord of fifth cusp Mars is occupied in third cusp is also in quincunx with Rahu indicates functional disorders related with uterus or ovaries. Saturn generally if afflicted with Uranus with sign Scorpio causes obstructive and inflammatory disorders with organ ruled by the cusp; in this case it is uterus and ovaries. The native when first visited in August 2005 for frequent menstruation problems, when asked to visit Doctor and got examined was found suffering from recurrent bladder infection and increased menstrual cramping with severe abdominal pain sometimes reported to have abnormal or heavy vaginal bleeding. When doctor examined her with diagnostic tests confirmed hyperactive thyroid gland and cysts developed in wall of uterus. So also, fallopian tubes were found blocked due to Pelvic Inflammation Disease.

According to KP system also it can be revealed that Star lord of ascendant Saturn which is also lord of eighth cusp occupied in fifth cusp and star lord of sixth cusp Ketu is placed in fourth house under aspect of Rahu which is star lord of twelfth cusp. Also, star lord of eighth house Mars is placed in third cusp conjoined with sub lord of ascendant Venus, which is also sub lord of fifth cusp. Sub lord of sixth cusp Saturn which is also sub lord of Saturn is placed in fifth cusp afflicted with Uranus. Sub lord of eighth cusp Moon is occupied in ninth house in quincunx with Ketu placed in fourth cusp. As such ascendant, sixth cusp, eighth cusp and twelfth cusp are well connected and indicates uterine functional and structural disorders.

The native was not required to get operated for hysterectomy and was totally recovered by curetting and medication. It was also evident that native had to suffer infertility even after applying modern latest techniques like IUI, followed by IVF but couldn't get conceived due to structural damages caused. Although doctors could save her uterus, she remained issueless. In this case simple infection caused initially if not attended in time and not noticed led to permanent infertility. Specifically, Jupiter which is lord of sixth cusp occupied in seventh cusp has played a crucial role in creating complications and as such in birth charts Jupiter, lord of sixth or eighth cusp and seventh house must be studied.

Planetary longitudes and disposition are tabled as below.

| Planets | Zodiac | Degrees | Lord of Zodiac | Star Lord | Sub Lord |
|---|---|---|---|---|---|
| Sun | Libra | 099:38:26 | Venus | Jupiter | Rahu |
| Moon | Pisces | 258:22:06 | Jupiter | Merc. | Mer |
| Mars | Virgo | 065:48:33 | Mercury | Sun | Mercury |
| Mercury | Libra | 119:50:36 | Venus | Jupiter | Moon |
| Jupiter | Capricorn | 194:21:28 | Saturn | Moon | Jupiter |
| Venus | Virgo | 079:03:29 | Mercury | Moon | Mercury |
| Saturn | Scorpio | 123:52:17 | Mars | Saturn | Saturn |
| Rahu | Aries | 285:40:25 | Mars | Venus | Sun |
| Ketu | Libra | 105:40:25 | Venus | Rahu | Venus |
| Uranus | Scorpio | 142:00:20 | Mars | Merc | Sun |
| Neptune | Sagittarius | 157:43:23 | Jupiter | Ketu | Jupiter |

## KP House Divisions and Lords of Cusp

| Cusp | Zodiac | Lord of Zodiac | Star Lord | Sub Lord |
|---|---|---|---|---|
| 01 | Cancer | Moon | Saturn | Venus |
| 02 | Leo | Sun | Ketu | Rahu |
| 03 | Virgo | Mercury | Sun | Mercury |
| 04 | Libra | Venus | Rahu | Rahu |
| 05 | Scorpio | Mars | Saturn | Venus |
| 06 | Sagittarius | Jupiter | Ketu | Saturn |
| 07 | Capricorn | Saturn | Moon | Moon |
| 08 | Aquarius | Saturn | Mars | Moon |
| 09 | Pisces | Jupiter | Saturn | Mercury |
| 10 | Aries | Mars | Ketu | Jupiter |
| 11 | Taurus | Venus | Moon | Moon |
| 12 | Gemini | Mercury | Rahu | Saturn |

Case No. 015/ssv
Date of birth 03rd July 1988 at 10:45 hours. In Hukkeri Karnataka with
Lat. 016:12 N Long. 074:36 E

In this Leo ascendant chart lord of ascendant placed in eleventh cusp under aspect of Mars occupied in eighth cusp, ascendant is occupied with Ketu and gives an indication of poor resistance or poor immunity to fight with odds. Ketu aspect Moon which is lord of twelfth house placed in seventh house with sign Aquarius denotes functional disorders of hormonal and lymph node system that causes Amenorrhea and poor immunity. Further lord of sixth cusp and seventh cusp Saturn is occupied in fifth cusp afflicted with Uranus and Neptune ascertains the structural and functional disorders of uterus, in this case it indicates mysterious malfunctioning of ovaries as indicated by Amenorrhea and serious abdominal pain cause for which becomes difficult to find. Also, Saturn aspect Sun placed in eleventh cusp which is lord of ascendant causing cranky mood or frequent mood swing and reduced strength to fight with odds. Mars which is lord of fourth cusp and ninth cusp is occupied in eighth cusp and in quadrant with Saturn causes growth of cyst in ovaries and may lead to serious pelvic inflammatory disorder that also blocks the fallopian tubes. Lord of third house and tenth house Venus is placed in tenth house conjoined with Jupiter which is lord of eighth cusp and Mercury indicates affected levels of hormone Follicle Stimulating Hormone and Antimulerian hormone which are responsible for smooth functioning of Menstruation cycle and function of ovaries. As also seventh house is afflicted with lord of fourth house Moon and Rahu indicates serious disorders related to hormonal imbalance and secretions of thyroid gland. If not attended in time this may cause permanent infertility. When in month of May 2018 native was asked to take help of expert Gynaecologist it was revealed that malfunctioning of thyroid associated with structural disorders related to Ovaries and uterus.

According to KP system also it can be understood clearly that the disorders related to ovaries and malfunctioning of thyroid are the cause of suffering. Star lord of ascendant Venus is conjoined with star lord of eighth cusp Mercury which is also star lord of twelfth cusp in tenth house in quadrant with Moon which is star lord of sixth cusp. Further Sub lord of ascendant Jupiter occupied in tenth cusp with sub lord of sixth cusp and eighth cusp Venus. Sub lord of twelfth cusp Sun is placed in eleventh house with sign Gemini lord of which is Mercury occupied in tenth cusp is also star lord twelfth cusp. This indicates ascendant; sixth cusp, eighth cusp and twelfth cusp are well connected gives serious disorders of reproductive system.

As said earlier the amenorrhea and abdominal pains reported in the month of May 2018 when Mahadasha of Jupiter was in progress and antardasha of Venus with pratiantardasha of Moon was appeared. In this case Moon is star lord of sixth cusp and Venus is sublord of sixth cusp.

It is also recommended that if the birth chart is studied for each woman entering adolescence many problems will be revealed much before they occur instead of waiting for marriage to take place and then visiting doctors for infertility issues which actually is outcome of uterine disorder. It is therefore may be envisaged to even every literate to understand even small problems related to uterine dysfunction and take timely advise of Experts to avoid further complications.

## Planetary longitudes and disposition

| Planet | Zodiac | Degrees | Lord of Zodiac | Star Lord | Sub Lord |
|---|---|---|---|---|---|
| Sun | Gemini | 317:47:41 | Mercury | Rahu | Sun |
| Moon | Aquarius | 184:17:31 | Saturn | Mars | Venus |
| Mars | Pisces | 211:04:25 | Jupiter | Jupiter | Mars |
| Mercury | Taurus | 297:11:15 | Venus | Mars | Jupiter |
| Jupiter | Taurus | 272:48:00 | Venus | Sun | Jupiter |
| Venus | Taurus | 230:15:59 | Venus | Moon | Ketu |
| Saturn | Sagittarius | 124:37:25 | Jupiter | Ketu | Moon |
| Rahu | Aquarius | 203:42:49 | Saturn | Jupiter | Saturn |
| Ketu | Leo | 023:42:49 | Sun | Venus | Saturn |
| Uranus | Sagittarius | 124:49:54 | Jupiter | Ketu | Mars |
| Neptune | Sagittarius | 135:02:23 | Jupiter | Venus | Venus |

## KP House Divisions and Lords of Cup

| Cusp | Zodiac | Lord of Zodiac | Star Lord | Sub Lord |
|---|---|---|---|---|
| 01 | Leo | Sun | Venus | Jupiter |
| 02 | Virgo | Mercury | Moon | Venus |
| 03 | Libra | Venus | Jupiter | Saturn |
| 04 | Scorpio | Mars | Mercury | Moon |
| 05 | Sagittarius | Jupiter | Venus | Saturn |
| 06 | Capricorn | Saturn | Moon | Venus |

| Cusp | Zodiac | Lord of Zodiac | Star Lord | Sub Lord |
|------|--------|----------------|-----------|----------|
| 07 | Aquarius | Saturn | Jupiter | Jupiter |
| 08 | Pisces | Jupiter | Mercury | Venus |
| 09 | Aries | Mars | Venus | Saturn |
| 10 | Taurus | Venus | Moon | Venus |
| 11 | Gemini | Mercury | Jupiter | Saturn |
| 12 | Cancer | Moon | Mercury | Sun |

Case No. 016/vk

Native born on 14th September 1983 at 19:22 hrs in Thane (West) with Lat 019:12 N Long 072:05 E

This is classic case of infertility syndrome due to complications of infection followed by functional disorders. The Pisces ascendant chart with lord of ascendant Jupiter is placed in ninth house afflicted with Uranus and Ketu; Jupiter is also lord of tenth house. Lord of second house and eighth cusp Mars is occupied in fifth cusp conjoined with lord of eighth cusp and third cusp Venus. Mars and Venus are under aspect of Saturn placed in eighth cusp which is lord of eleventh and twelfth cusp. Lord of fifth cusp Moon is placed in tenth house afflicted with Neptune and under aspect of Saturn occupied in eighth cusp, which indicates hormonal disorders and function of ovaries. Also, Sun which is lord of sixth cusp is occupied in sixth cusp conjoined with lord of fourth cusp and seventh cusp indicating functional disorders like secretary function of ovaries causing frequent abnormal vaginal bleeding and pain in pelvic region or lower belly. Also, it is noticed that native suffers painful menstrual periods. Further it can be observed that Mercury being lord of seventh house conjoined with lord of sixth cusp in sixth cusp causes endometriosis which also is likely to add to pain during periods. Native when approached doctor for examination and treatment it was diagnosed that the cause of suffering is hyper prolactenemia and polycystic ovarian syndrome.

Also, the native was suffering from folic acid deficiency syndrome. According to KP system also it can be clarified that as star lord of ascendant Saturn is placed in eighth cusp in quincunx with Rahu which is star lord of eighth cusp. Further star lord of twelfth cusp is occupied in fifth cusp under aspect of Saturn. Sub lord of ascendant Sun is placed in sixth cusp with sub lord of eighth cusp Mercury and in quincunx with Moon which is sub lord of sixth cusp; Venus which is sub lord of eighth cusp is also sub lord of twelfth cusp.

Thus ascendant, sixth house, eighth cusp and twelfth cusp are well connected indicating severe functional disorders associated with uterus and ovaries.

The occurrence of the disease first noticed in the month of October 2015 when native suffered extreme abdominal pain and irregular menstruation. Native was got recovered from the disease after prolonged medical treatment by experts in the month of March 2019.

Planetary longitudes and disposition as detailed in table below.

| Planet | Zodiac | Degrees | Lord of Zodiac | StarLord | Sub Lord |
|---|---|---|---|---|---|
| Sun | Leo | 177:33:23 | Sun | Sun | Moon |
| Moon | Sagittarius | 272:58:20 | Jupiter | Ketu | Venus |
| Mars | Cancer | 146:43:12 | Moon | Mercury | Jupiter |
| Mercury | Leo | 179:43:59 | Saturn | Sun | Rahu |
| Jupiter | Scorpio | 250:39:23 | Mars | Saturn | Sun |
| Venus | Cancer | 149:36:10 | Moon | Merc | Saturn |
| Saturn | Libra | 218:17:29 | Venus | Rahu | Rahu |
| Rahu | Taurus | 086:38:54 | Venus | Mars | Jupiter |
| Ketu | Scorpio | 266:38:54 | Mars | Merc | Jupiter |
| Uranus | Scorpio | 251:51:49 | Mars | Saturn | Moon |
| Neptune | Sagittarius | 272:50:55 | Jupiter | Ketu | Venus |

## KP House Divisions and Lords of Cusp

| Cusp | Zodiac | Lord of Zodiac | Star Lord | SubLord |
|---|---|---|---|---|
| 01 | Pisces | Jupiter | Saturn | Sun |
| 02 | Aries | Mars | Venus | Venus |
| 03 | Taurus | Venus | Moon | Jupiter |
| 04 | Gemini | Mercury | Rahu | Jupiter |
| 05 | Cancer | Moon | Saturn | Saturn |
| 06 | Leo | Sun | Ketu | Moon |
| 07 | Virgo | Mercury | Moon | Moon |
| 08 | Libra | Venus | Rahu | Venus |
| 09 | Scorpio | Mars | Saturn | Rahu |
| 10 | Sagittarius | Jupiter | Ketu | Jupiter |
| 11 | Capricorn | Saturn | Sun | Saturn |
| 12 | Aquarius | Saturn | Mars | Venus |

Case No. 017/bsr
Native born on 19ᵗʰ February 1982 at16:40 hours in Nasik with
Lat. 020:00 N Long. 073:48 E

This is Cancer ascendant chart with lord of ascendant Moon occupied in sixth cusp afflicted with Ketu and Neptune indicating functional problems related to hormones and especially thyroxin hormone. Also, lord of second house Leo is occupied in eighth cusp with sign Aquarius indicates poor immunity with poor strength to fight with diseases. Lord of third house and twelfth house Mercury is occupied in seventh cusp conjoined with Venus which is lord of third and eleventh cusp indicating disorders related to reproductive system especially as the conjunction occupied in Aquarius it is indicated that functional disorders of uterus and ovaries. Jupiter which is lord of sixth house and ninth house is placed in fourth cusp with sign Libra also denotes the uterine abnormalities. Lord of fifth cusp and tenth cusp Mars is placed in third house afflicted with Saturn which is lord of eighth cusp and seventh cusp indicates obstructive and inflammatory chronic disorders of uterus. Also, it is seen that Saturn aspect fifth house causing obstructive growth either in uterus or in ovaries. In this case Sun occupied in eighth cusp with sign Aquarius also gives cranky and irritating type of mood associated with uncontrollable anger causing secretion of catecholamines in body that causes further complications of uterine function which is noticed specifically when the dysfunctional bleeding during two menstrual cycle occurs. Also, this Sun is likely to give obesity disorder due to voracious eating habits giving unwanted weight gain that further causes disturbed function of uterus. When the native approached for getting horoscope studied and solution to this problem was first asked to consult Gynecologist for thorough examination of pelvis and accordingly doctor conducted few tests like FSH, LH, and Prolactin it was evident that the uterus has benign neoplasm and ectopic growth of endometrial tissue within myometrium. Doctors also noticed the hyperactive thyroid with high levels of TSH that might have caused weight gain. Doctor advised to go for surgical removal of the benign growth and given certain medicines for TSH.

According to KP system also we can confirm this; as star lord of ascendant Saturn is placed in third house with Sign Virgo. Sixth cusp conjoined with sub lord of ascendant Moon and under aspect of star lord of eighth cusp Rahu which is also lord of twelfth cusp. Sub lord of sixth cusp Mercury is occupied in seventh house in quincunx with Rahu which is sub lord of eighth cusp with sign Capricorn owned by Saturn which is sub lord of twelfth house indicating the ascendant, sixth cusp, eighth cusp, and twelfth cusp are well connected giving rise to the complicated uterine functional and structural disorders. The occurrence of the disease was actually noticed due to dysfunctional bleeding occurred during two menstrual cycles in the month of March 2011 but it appears that the growth of the disease must have started much earlier. In March 2011 Moon mahadasha was in progress with Ketu antardasha and pratiantardasha of also Ketu.

Native got recovered after surgical removal of benign growth leaving behind the scar and permanent infertility.

## Planetary longitudes and disposition chart

| Planet | Zodiac | Degrees | Lord of Zodiac | Star Lord | Sub Lord |
| --- | --- | --- | --- | --- | --- |
| Sun | Aquarius | 216:52:33 | Saturn | Rahu | Rahu |
| Moon | Sagittarius | 166:07:09 | Jupiter | Venus | Sun |
| Mars | Virgo | 085:33:55 | Mercury | Mars | Rahu |
| Mercury | Capricorn | 191:18:17 | Saturn | Moon | Mars |
| Jupiter | Libra | 106:41:18 | Venus | Rahu | Venus |
| Venus | Capricorn | 181:10:59 | Saturn | Sun | Rahu |
| Saturn | Virgo | 088:19:08 | Mercury | Mars | Saturn |
| Rahu | Gemini | 356:57:55 | Mercury | Jupiter | Venus |
| Ketu | Sagittarius | 176:57:55 | Jupiter | Sun | Sun |
| Uranus | Scorpio | 130:52:14 | Mars | Saturn | Sun |
| Neptune | Sagittarius | 153:02:16 | Jupiter | Ketu | Sun |

## KP House Divisions and Lords of Cusp

| Cusp | Zodiac | Lord of Zodiac | Star Lord | Sub Lord |
| --- | --- | --- | --- | --- |
| 01 | Cancer | Moon | Saturn | Moon |
| 02 | Leo | Sun | Ketu | Jupiter |
| 03 | Virgo | Mercury | Sun | Mercury |
| 04 | Libra | Venus | Rahu | Jupiter |
| 05 | Scorpio | Mars | Saturn | Moon |
| 06 | Sagittarius | Jupiter | Ketu | Mercury |
| 07 | Capricorn | Saturn | Moon | Mars |
| 08 | Aquarius | Saturn | Rahu | Rahu |

| Cusp | Zodiac | Lord of Zodiac | Star Lord | Sub Lord |
|---|---|---|---|---|
| 09 | Pisces | Jupiter | Saturn | Mercury |
| 10 | Aries | Mars | Ketu | Jupiter |
| 11 | Taurus | Venus | Moon | Mars |
| 12 | Gemini | Mercury | Rahu | Saturn |

Case No. 018/psd

Native born on 23rd May 1991 at 12:28 hours in Dhulia

Lat. 020:54 N Long. 074:47 E

This chart with Leo ascendant is classic chart indicating complex uterine problems. Lord of ascendant Sun is occupied in tenth house with sign Taurus placed in quadrant with Saturn occupied in sixth house as lord of sixth house and seventh cusp, this causes repeated ovarian malfunction with frequent infection. Further lord of second house Mercury which rules the structural and functional disorders of uterine wall and ovaries is placed in ninth cusp with sign Aries lord of which is occupied in twelfth cusp. Also Moon which rules secretary function of ovaries and Thyroid is placed in second cusp with sign Virgo; Mercury is lord of twelfth cusp lord of fourth cusp Mars is occupied in twelfth cusp conjoined with Jupiter which is lord of fifth cusp and eighth cusp denotes the disorders of ovaries with some abnormal growth of cells. Further fifth house is occupied by Uranus conjoined with Neptune and Rahu indicates serious malfunctioning of ovaries. Also, fifth house is under aspect of Ketu placed in eleventh house afflicting Venus which is lord of tenth cusp and rules the functioning of reproductive system. It can be observed that lord of fifth cusp and eighth cusp Jupiter is under aspect of Saturn occupied with own sign Capricorn in sixth house which rules the various disorders and diseases of body. Again, Saturn being lord of seventh house occupied in sixth cusp also indicates the malfunctioning of reproductive system. When native approached for seeking solution when marriage will take place was advised first to consult doctor and was suffering from severe pain in abdomen during periods associated with irregular periods and other problems which were ignored previously. After examination doctor advised certain drugs to overcome problem and advised curetting of uterus. The actual onset of this problem started long back in 2007 somewhere but totally ignored as it is routine of female life; and, got appropriately treated by doctors in 2018. According to KP system also it can be seen that afflicted fifth house has caused the problem. Star lord of ascendant Ketu is occupied in eleventh house conjoined with Venus which is sub lord of sixth cusp. Also, star lord of sixth cusp Sun is placed in tenth house in quincunx with Rahu sub lord of eleventh house aspect ketu which is star lord of fifth cusp. Further star lord of twelfth house Saturn which is also star lord of eighth cusp is occupied in sixth cusp aspect sub lord of ascendant Jupiter placed in twelfth cusp. Sub lord of eighth cusp Mercury is placed in ninth house in quadrant with Saturn which is star lord of eighth and twelfth house. Sub lord of sixth house and twelfth house Venus is placed in eleventh house is also in quincunx with Saturn. All this indicate the afflicted and debilitated fifth house that caused serious functional disorders associated with uterus and ovaries. The date of actual occurrence of the disease is not exactly recorded but it appears to be in mahadasha of Mars with antardasha of Venus in the month of April 2007 as per the discussion with native.

## Planetary longitudes and disposition

| Planet | Zodiac | Degrees | Lord of Zodiac | Star Lord | Sub Lord |
| --- | --- | --- | --- | --- | --- |
| Sun | Taurus | 277:55:36 | Venus | Sun | Venus |
| Moon | Virgo | 038:20:06 | Mercury | Sun | Venus |
| Mars | Cancer | 334:22:39 | Moon | Saturn | Saturn |
| Mercury | Aries | 254:33:39 | Mars | Venus | Venus |
| Jupiter | Cancer | 343:56:56 | Moon | Saturn | Rahu |
| Venus | Gemini | 321:54:10 | Mercury | Jupiter | Saturn |
| Saturn | Capricorn | 163:04:15 | Saturn | Moon | Rahu |
| Rahu | Sagitta | 147:51:12 | Jupiter | Sun | Moon |
| Ketu | Gemini | 327:51:12 | Mercury | Jupiter | Venus |
| Uranus | Sagitta | 139:35:19 | Jupiter | Venus | Rahu |
| Neptune | Sagitta | 142:43:09 | Jupiter | Venus | Saturn |

## KP House Divisions and Lords of cusp

| Cusp | Zodiac | Lord of Zodiac | Star Lord | Sub Lord |
| --- | --- | --- | --- | --- |
| 01 | Leo | Sun | Ketu | Jupiter |
| 02 | Virgo | Mercury | Sun | Mercury |
| 03 | Libra | Venus | Mars | Moon |
| 04 | Scorpio | Mars | Saturn | Venus |
| 05 | Sagittarius | Jupiter | Ketu | Jupiter |

| Cusp | Zodiac | Lord of Zodiac | Star Lord | Sub Lord |
|---|---|---|---|---|
| 06 | Capricorn | Saturn | Sun | Venus |
| 07 | Aquarius | Saturn | Rahu | Rahu |
| 08 | Pisces | Jupiter | Saturn | Mercury |
| 09 | Aries | Mars | Ketu | Rahu |
| 10 | Taurus | Venus | Sun | Venus |
| 11 | Gemini | Mercury | Rahu | Jupiter |
| 12 | Cancer | Moon | Saturn | Venus |

Case No. 019/vyr

Native born on 30th March 1982 at 00:00 hours in Miraj
with Lat 016:49 N Long 074:38 E

This is a rare birth chart with Scorpio ascendant occupied by Uranus indicating mysterious diseases are likely to occur. Lord of ascendant Mars is occupied in eleventh house aspect the fifth house; Mars is also lord of sixth cusp. This causes abnormal growth in ovaries leading to PCOD (polycystic ovarian disorder). Further Venus which is lord of twelfth house and second house is placed in third cusp with sign Capricorn indicating inflammatory and infectious diseases of uterus. Also, fifth house is occupied by Sun with sign Pisces and conjoined with lord of eighth house and eleventh house Mercury which rules the tissue lining of uterus and uterine tract. Sun and Mercury are under aspect of Mars and as such causes repeated malfunctioning of ovaries. Saturn conjoined with Mars also aspect fifth cusp indicates obstructive and inflammatory diseases of uterus. Lord of ninth house Moon is occupied in seventh house is under aspect of Uranus placed in ascendant. This indicates severe infectious and inflammatory diseases of uterus and ovaries which causes functional disorders of ovaries and hormonal imbalance. Jupiter lord of fifth house is placed in twelfth house hemmed in between Uranus and Saturn leads to abnormal growth of cyst in uterus and ovaries. it is also can be noticed that Sun occupied in fifth house is in quadrant with Rahu placed in eighth house gives growth of cysts in ovaries. Native when visited me for delayed marriage and remedial measures for the same but when her horoscope was opened it is revealed instantly that there is problem associated with uterus and also was told by client regarding mild persistent pain in lower belly with frequent irregular menstrual periods the native was asked to consult expert doctor first. It was astonishing that doctor when diagnosed found polycystic ovarian growth in both the ovaries. One ovary was surgically removed and another was then treated with medication. This normally happens only because uterine health is always given secondary importance.

According to KP system also it can be confirmed that the uterus or ovaries is the cause of health issues. The star lord of ascendant Mercury is occupied in fifth house with Sun which is sub lord of eighth cusp and star lord of sixth house under aspect of Saturn which is star lord of twelfth cusp and in quincunx with Jupiter which is star lord of eighth house. Saturn is sub lord of ascendant, sixth house and twelfth house occupied in eleventh house with Mars which is lord of sixth cusp. Thus ascendant, sixth house, eighth house and twelfth house are well connected indicating debilitated fifth house that rules the uterus and ovaries. The occurrence of the disease was not exactly found but native was required to be hospitalized for surgical removal of ovary in the month of March 2012, when Mahadasha of Rahu was in progress with antardasha of Sun and pratiantardasha of Saturn was occurred. In this case Sun and Saturn is star lord of sixth house and sub lord of sixth house, respectively.

Planetary longitudes and disposition are tabled as under.

| Planet | Zodiac | Degrees | Lord of Zodiac | Star Lord | Sub Lord |
| --- | --- | --- | --- | --- | --- |
| Sun | Scorpio | 135:07:58 | Jupiter | Saturn | Jupiter |
| Moon | Pisces | 192:50:29 | Venus | Moon | Rahu |
| Mars | Taurus | 317:24:18 | Mercury | Moon | Saturn |
| Mercury | Virgo | 122:32:12 | Jupiter | Jupiter | Rahu |
| Jupiter | Pisces | 345:01:56 | Venus | Rahu | Ketu |
| Venus | Libra | 088:44:13 | Saturn | Mars | Saturn |
| Saturn | Capricorn | 326:06:07 | Mercury | Mars | Rahu |
| Rahu | Virgo | 234:56:09 | Mercury | Jupiter | Mercury |
| Ketu | Gemini | 054:56:09 | Jupiter | Venus | Mercury |
| Uranus | Sagittarius | 010:50:54 | Mars | Saturn | Sun |
| Neptune | Scorpio | 033:26:21 | Jupiter | Ketu | Sun |

KP House Divisions and Lords of Cusp

| Cusp | Zodiac | Lord of Zodiac | Star Lord | Sub Lord |
|------|--------|----------------|-----------|----------|
| 01 | Scorpio | Mars | Mercury | Saturn |
| 02 | Sagittarius | Jupiter | Sun | Mars |
| 03 | Aquarius | Saturn | Mars | Mercury |
| 04 | Pisces | Jupiter | Saturn | Saturn |
| 05 | Aries | Mars | Ketu | Rahu |
| 06 | Taurus | Venus | Sun | Saturn |
| 07 | Taurus | Venus | Mars | Saturn |
| 08 | Gemini | Mercury | Jupiter | Sun |
| 09 | Leo | Sun | Ketu | Venus |
| 10 | Virgo | Mercury | Sun | Mercury |
| 11 | Libra | Venus | Mars | Moon |
| 12 | Scorpio | Mars | Saturn | Saturn |

Case No. 020/ssd
Native born on 18<sup>th</sup> February 1988 at 20:05 hours in Pune with
Lat. 018:30 N Long. 073:48 E

In this chart with Leo ascendant and the lord of ascendant Sun is placed in seventh house with sign Aquarius and conjoined with Moon which is lord of twelfth house. This indicates the functional disorders associated with uterus and ovaries. Venus which rules the reproductive organs and lord of third and fourth cusp is occupied in eighth cusp afflicted with Rahu denotes the serious structural disorders of uterus. Further lord of second house Virgo and eleventh house Gemini Mercury is occupied in sixth cusp; as Mercury rules the epithelial and mucosal layers of uterus causes severe infection with affected secretary functions. in this chart it also can be seen that fifth house is occupied by Mars which is lord of fourth and ninth cusp afflicted with lord of sixth house Saturn which rules obstructive and chronic types of diseases. Uranus and Neptune are also occupied in fifth house with Mars and Saturn indicates mysterious difficult to diagnose diseases of uterus. Lord of fifth house Jupiter is placed in ninth house with sign Aries and as such indicates growth of abnormal cells. This is very interesting to understand the effect of Saturn when it becomes lord of sixth and seventh cusp and occupies fifth cusp as it not only creates structural disorders but also produces long lasting negative impact on the uterine health.

In this case it is noticeable that initially in the month of May year 2002 caused severe inflammation with growth of multiple cysts and was recovered in 2004 January. Again, the same thing appeared in 2015 after marriage creating threat of permanent infertility and again got recovered which relapsed in July 2019 after birth of first child. The cause of repetitive occurrence of the growth of cysts in ovaries and in the wall of uterus was certainly mystery for doctors. As it is seen in the chart that Moon being lord of twelfth house occupies seventh house some functional disorders were noticed also mild hyperthyroidism was also noticed but the major effect of Saturn, Mars, Uranus and Neptune if fifth house with sign Sagittarius was distinguished and was difficult to diagnose. It appears uterine health after menopause will be worse.

According to KP system star lord of ascendant Sun is placed in seventh house afflicted with lord of twelfth house. Star lord of sixth house Mars is occupied in fifth house with Uranus and Neptune. Lord of eighth cusp Mercury which is also star lord of twelfth house is placed in sixth house owned by Saturn. Further sub lord of ascendant Sun occupied in seventh house in triangle with Jupiter which is sub lord of sixth, eighth and twelfth cusp. This indicates severe infectious growth of cells in uterus and ovaries. The first occurrence of the disease as indicated by absence of periods for more than three months with acute pains in the abdomen was noticed in May 2002 when Jupiter mahadasha was in progress and antardasha and pratiantardasha of Mars was continued. Where the Jupiter is sub lord of sixth cusp and Mars is star lord of sixth cusp.

Planetary longitudes and disposition is tabled as under.

| Planet | Zodiac | Degrees | Lord of Zodiac | Star Lord | Sub Lord |
| --- | --- | --- | --- | --- | --- |
| Sun | Aquarius | 185:28:00 | Saturn | Mars | Sun |
| Moon | Aquarius | 198:52:07 | Saturn | Rahu | Moon |
| Mars | Sagittarius | 123:44:13 | Jupiter | Ketu | Moon |
| Mercury | Capricorn | 170:34:42 | Saturn | Moon | Venus |
| Jupiter | Aries | 242:35:26 | Mars | Ketu | Venus |
| Venus | Pisces | 226:59:42 | Jupiter | Merc | Mercury |
| Saturn | Sagittarius | 126:41:08 | Jupiter | Ketu | Rahu |
| Rahu | Pisces | 210:54:01 | Jupiter | Jupiter | Mars |
| Ketu | Virgo | 030:54:01 | Mercury | Sun | Rahu |
| Uranus | Sagittarius | 126:26:55 | Jupiter | Ketu | Rahu |
| Neptune | Sagittarius | 135:45:03 | Jupiter | Venus | Sun |

## KP House Divisions and Lords of cusp

| Cusp | Zodiac | Lord of Zodiac | Star Lord | Sub Lord |
|---|---|---|---|---|
| 01 | Leo | Sun | Sun | Sun |
| 02 | Virgo | Mercury | Mars | Jupiter |
| 03 | Libra | Venus | Jupiter | Venus |
| 04 | Scorpio | Mars | Mercury | Jupiter |
| 05 | Sagittarius | Jupiter | Sun | Moon |
| 06 | Capricorn | Saturn | Mars | Jupiter |
| 07 | Aquarius | Saturn | Jupiter | Venus |
| 08 | Pisces | Jupiter | Mercury | Jupiter |
| 09 | Aries | Mars | Sun | Sun |
| 10 | Taurus | Venus | Mars | Jupiter |
| 11 | Gemini | Mercury | Jupiter | Venus |
| 12 | Cancer | Moon | Mercury | Jupiter |

# Chapter 5

# Complications of Conception and Subs

In pregnancy sometimes complications are observed are either because of previous history, malnutrition or other congenital history in family. The major complications include Pregnancy hypertension, pregnancy diabetes or history of congenital disabilities in family related to genetic problems. If woman or partner or close family member have genetic abnormalities or have given birth to a child with congenital disabilities are at higher risk of miscarriage or pregnancy complications. Also, addictions like smoking, consuming alcohol, cocaine, high levels of caffeine, etc. also causes pregnancy complications.

Diabetes in pregnancy or hypertension in pregnancy is mostly occurred complications amongst others. As already discussed earlier few examples who have specifically contacted for guidance are enclosed herewith for further study.

Case No. 021/mpc
Date of birth 31ˢᵗ July 1979 at 10:30 hours. in Mumbai/ Santacruz
Lat. 019:05 N Long. 072:50 E

Virgo ascendant chart with lord of ascendant Mercury is placed in eleventh house conjoined with Venus, Jupiter and Sun. Lord of fifth cusp Saturn is placed in twelfth cusp Afflicted with Rahu indicating obstructive disorders related to uterus. Ketu is occupied in sixth cusp with sign Aquarius aspect the Saturn causing inflammatory disorders of uterus. Lord of eighth cusp and third cusp Mars is occupied in tenth house with sign Gemini. This indicates blood related functional disorders, also as Mars aspect fifth cusp and itself is under aspect of Saturn causes pregnancy complications especially related to blood. Venus which rules functions of uterus and ovaries is hemmed in between Saturn and Mars indicates premature delivery or difficulty in delivery. Sun which is lord of twelfth house aspect the fifth house indicates the functional disorders of uterus during pregnancy especially related to the cardiac activity of fetus in womb. Jupiter which rules the overall growth is also hemmed in between Saturn and Mars causes congenital development problems in pregnancy. Mercury which rules the nerve supply to uterus and epithelial lining of uterus gives an indication of some or other structural problems associated with growing fetus. Considering all this together it can be revealed that pregnancy for this native is not normal and some complications are likely to take place and as such were advised to consult another Gynecologist for second opinion. When the native was subjected to ultra-sonography once again it was observed that native was suffering from Oligohydramnios which means low amniotic fluid leading to malnutrition of fetus. This was cause because of leaking or ruptured membranes and problems with placenta. Doctors tried their level best but due to low amniotic fluid they must advise premature induced delivery. Naturally, this was shock to mother but there were no options before. The infant being suffered from malnutrition and found to have developmental problems with kidneys could not be saved. In this case each doctor had taken every care till end but problems were developed unnoticing and were beyond the reach of treatment. The occurrence of the incidence was noticed in the month of December 2014 when Jupiter mahadasha was in progress and antardasha of Rahu with pratiantardasha of Mercury occurred. Where Mercury is sub lord of sixth cusp and Rahu is star lord of sixth cusp.

According to KP system also it can be observed that fifth house and pregnancy complications were to occur. Star lord of ascendant is Moon placed in second house under aspect of Saturn which is afflicted with Rahu, star lord of sixth house. Also, star lord of eighth cusp Ketu which is also star lord of twelfth cusp is placed in sixth house under aspect of Rahu. Rahu is also sub lord of ascendant indicates complications while in pregnancy are expected. Further Mercury, which is sub lord of sixth, eighth house, and twelfth cusp is placed in eleventh house aspect the fifth cusp and hemmed in between Saturn and Mars causes premature delivery. As such ascendant, sixth cusp, eighth house and twelfth cusp are well connected and indicate the problems associated with baby birth.

Thus, it is noticeably clear to understand that birth chart is indicating the complications during pregnancy before they were occurred. The period of occurrence as referred above can be understood to be between the Dasha periods of lords of sixth house.

It is therefore can be recommended that even though native is under treatment with expert doctor shall approach for second opinion in order to eliminate black spot that may remain in the observation of known doctors.

Planetary longitudes and disposition for case no. 021/mpc

| Planet | Zodiac | Degrees | Lord of Zodiac | Star Lord | Sub Lord |
|---|---|---|---|---|---|
| Sun | Cancer | 313:50:42 | Moon | Saturn | Rahu |
| Moon | Libra | 031:56:01 | Venus | Mars | Ketu |
| Mars | Gemini | 270:49:59 | Mercury | Mars | Mercury |
| Merc | Cancer | 314:43:48 | Moon | Saturn | Rahu |
| Jupiter. | Cancer | 323:34:49 | Moon | Mercury | Mars |
| Venus | Cancer | 306:53:10 | Moon | Saturn | Mercury |
| Saturn | Leo | 348:41:45 | Sun | Venus | Rahu |
| Rahu | Leo | 346:28:15 | Sun | Venus | Moon |
| Ketu | Aquarius. | 136:28:15 | Saturn | Rahu | Venus |
| Uranus | Libra | 053:21:35 | Venus | Jupiter | Saturn |
| Neptune | Scorpio | 084:23:28 | Mars | Mercury | Rahu |

## KP House Divisions and Lords of Cusp

| Cusp | Zodiac | Lord of Zodiac | Star Lord | Sub Lord |
|---|---|---|---|---|
| 01 | Virgo | Mercury | Moon | Rahu |
| 02 | Libra | Venus | Rahu | Saturn |
| 03 | Scorpio | Mars | Saturn | Moon |
| 04 | Sagittarius | Jupiter | Ketu | Mercury |
| 05 | Capricorn | Saturn | Moon | Rahu |
| 06 | Aquarius | Saturn | Rahu | Mercury |
| 07 | Pisces | Jupiter | Saturn | Mars |
| 08 | Aries | Mars | Ketu | Mercury |
| 09 | Taurus | Venus | Moon | Rahu |
| 10 | Gemini | Mercury | Rahu | Saturn |
| 11 | Cancer | Moon | Saturn | Mars |
| 12 | Leo | Sun | Ketu | Mercury |

Case No. 022/sdm
Date of birth 26th April 1990 at 11:50 hours in Khanapur with
Lat. 015:39 N Long. 074:31 E

Cancer ascendant chart with lord of ascendant Moon is occupied in twelfth house indicates blood related disorders. Mon is conjoined with Jupiter which is lord of sixth cusp as such also indicates functional disorders of secondary reproductive system, also Jupiter and Moon are in quincunx with Saturn afflicted with Rahu and occupied in seventh house denotes frequent miscarriages. Jupiter and Moon are also under aspect of Uranus and Neptune which are known to cause mysterious diseases that lead to miscarriage. Lord of fifth cusp is placed in eighth house with sign Aquarius causes spontaneous abortion due to under or no development of cardiac activity in fetus even beyond 16th week of pregnancy. It was in the month of January 2016 i. e. after eleventh week of pregnancy according to doctor was just completed, it was observed in the birth chart about abortion of pregnancy the native was asked to consult their expert doctor immediately. After the thorough medical examination and USG tests it was diagnosed by doctor that there are no symptoms of cardiac activity and after waiting for a week further was advised to abort the pregnancy. This was also observed that the native was not at all having any family history of abortions or miscarriages neither the native was having any history of hypertension or trauma stress earlier to abortions. The reason behind inactive cardiac could not have been diagnosed. It was probable related to blood disorders which were not noticed during the period. Further the native was not having any addictions or bad habits or family stress that might have caused the problem. Doctors could not give any reason for this kind of absence of cardiac activity.

According to KP system also it is noticed that star lord of ascendant Saturn is placed in seventh house afflicted with Rahu, star lord of twelfth house and aspect Ketu which is star lord sixth cusp and in quincunx with Mars which is star lord of eighth house. Sub lord of ascendant Mercury occupied in tenth house placed in quadrant with Rahu, sub lord of sixth house which is also sub lord of twelfth house. Rahu is occupied in seventh house conjoined with Saturn and aspect Venus occupied in ninth house. As such ascendant, sixth house, eighth house and twelfth house are well connected indicating the miscarriage and suffering of native. The native approached Doctor on January 5th, 2016 for second opinion as advised and then operated for curetting on

January 9th, 2016. During this period mahadasha of Jupiter and antardasha of Rahu with just started Pratiantardasha of Ketu was in progress. Rahu is sub lord of sixth cusp and Ketu is star lord of sixth cusp.

It is worth noting here that the health of native was exceptionally good and age of nearing thirty is also not risky. There was no history of miscarriages in family or even there was no congenital disorders and thus exact cause of under development of heart in fetus is not known.

It is assumed that because of low amniotic fluid or some congenital problems or may be because of chromosomal disorders associated with mother. It is also worth noting that the even in absence of history of any congenital problems like this the cardiac development could not take place.

## Planetary Longitudes and disposition

| Planet | Zodiac | Degrees | Lord of Zodiac | Star Lord | Sub Lord |
|---|---|---|---|---|---|
| Sun | Aries | 284:57:29 | Mars | Venus | Venus |
| Moon | Gemini | 342:04:30 | Mercury | Rahu | Saturn |
| Mars | Aquarius | 222:30:43 | Saturn | Rahu | Saturn |
| Mercury | Aries | 292:16:14 | Mars | Venus | Saturn |
| Jupiter | Gemini | 342:55:36 | Mercury | Rahu | Mercury |
| Venus | Pisces | 240:49:14 | Jupiter | Jupiter | Mars |
| Saturn | Capricorn | 181:35:16 | Saturn | Sun | Jupiter |
| Rahu | Capricorn | 198:28:10 | Saturn | Moon | Mercury |
| Ketu | Cancer | 018:28:10 | Moon | Mercury | Mercury |
| Uranus | Sagittarius | 165:45:56 | Jupiter | Venus | Sun |
| Neptune | Sagittarius | 170:48:21 | Jupiter | Venus | Jupiter |

## KP House Divisions and Lord of cusp

| Cusp | Zodiac | Lord of Zodiac | Star Lord | Sub Lord |
|---|---|---|---|---|
| 01 | Cancer | Moon | Saturn | Mercury |
| 02 | Leo | Sun | Ketu | Sun |
| 03 | Virgo | Mercury | Sun | Jupiter |
| 04 | Libra | Venus | Mars | Venus |
| 05 | Scorpio | Mars | Saturn | Mercury |
| 06 | Sagittarius | Jupiter | Ketu | Rahu |
| 07 | Capricorn | Saturn | Sun | Mercury |
| 08 | Aquarius | Saturn | Mars | Venus |

| Cusp | Zodiac | Lord of Zodiac | Star Lord | Sub Lord |
|------|--------|----------------|-----------|----------|
| 09 | Pisces | Jupiter | Jupiter | Rahu |
| 10 | Aries | Mars | Ketu | Mars |
| 11 | Taurus | Venus | Sun | Mercury |
| 12 | Gemini | Mercury | Rahu | Rahu |

Case No. 023/ kyp

Date of Birth26[th]March 1988 at 12:00 hours in Pune

Lat. 018:38 N Long. 073:48 E

This is classic Gemini ascendant chart with lord of ascendant Mercury occupied in ninth house with sign Aquarius and afflicted with Rahu. Mercury is also under aspect of Saturn placed in seventh house which is lord of eighth and ninth house and as such indicates gestational hypertension that leads to preeclampsia. Further Moon which rules the function of uterus and hormones is occupied in tenth house conjoined with Sun lord of third house is in quincunx with Ketu occupied in third house. Mars which is lord of sixth cusp and eleventh cusp is occupied in seventh house afflicted with Saturn, lord of eighth and eleventh house and Uranus with Neptune. This causes pregnancy hypertension. Jupiter which is lord of seventh house and tenth house indicates healthy growth of fetus as it is conjoined with Venus which is lord of fifth house also Venus is lord of twelfth house is likely to cause painful delivery of child and may also cause threat to mother's health. As seventh house is occupied with Uranus which is known for mysterious diseases cause protein in urine with hypertension called preeclampsia.

The native when visited for understanding the horoscope reading of mother and child it was noticed that some ailments are there which are likely to cause delivery painful and native may have family history of hypertension. Therefore, advised to revisit doctor and seek his opinion regarding this. Doctor when examined found blood pressure about 140/100 and asked native to consume some medications and to get it regularly monitored. It was further confirmed that though the fetus was healthy but because of native's health the delivery got complicate. As the blood pressure if shoots above 140/90 is likely to cause serious health threat to unborn baby it was necessary for doctors to treat it first which native didn't notice till visit to doctor. This requires induced labor during delivery. According to KP system also hospitalization due to hypertension is indicated. Star lord of ascendant Rahu is occupied in ninth house conjoined with Mercury under aspect of Saturn which is star lord of sixth cusp and placed at 30 degrees from Sun which is star lord of eighth and twelfth house. Sub lord of ascendant is Jupiter and is conjoined with sub lord of sixth and twelfth house. Sub lord of eighth cusp is Saturn occupied in seventh house aspect ascendant. As such Ascendant, sixth house, house, eighth house and twelfth house are well connected and denotes the complications related to pregnancy of native. The native delivered a healthy baby but acquired hypertension for lifetime during pregnancy.

## Planetary longitudes and disposition

| Planet | Zodiac | Degrees | Lord of Zodiac | Star Lord | Sub Lord |
|---|---|---|---|---|---|
| Sun | Pisces | 282:07:40 | Jupiter | Saturn | Mars |
| Moon | Pisces | 294:08:47 | Mercury | Jupiter | Mercury |
| Mars | Sagitta | 208:28:09 | Jupiter | Sun | Mars |
| Merc | Aquarius | 260:19:33 | Saturn | Jupiter | Jupiter |
| Jupiter | Aries | 310:08:18 | Mars | Ketu | Saturn |
| Venus | Aries | 327:47:45 | Mars | Sun | Moon |
| Saturn | Sagitta | 188:39:20 | Jupiter | Ketu | Jupiter |
| Rahu | Aquarius | 268:57:27 | Saturn | Jupiter | Sun |
| Ketu | Leo | 088:57:27 | Sun | Sun | Mars |
| Uranus | Sagittarius | 187:18:52 | Jupiter | Ketu | Rahu |

## KP House Divisions and Lords of Cusp

| Cusp | Zodiac | Lord of Zodiac | Star Lord | Sub Lord |
|---|---|---|---|---|
| 01 | Gemini | Mercury | Rahu | Jupiter |
| 02 | Cancer | Moon | Saturn | Saturn |
| 03 | Leo | Sun | Ketu | Venus |
| 04 | Virgo | Mercury | Sun | Rahu |
| 05 | Libra | Venus | Mars | Sun |
| 06 | Scorpio | Mars | Saturn | Venus |
| 07 | Sagittarius | Jupiter | Ketu | Saturn |
| 08 | Capricorn | Saturn | Sun | Saturn |
| 09 | Aquarius | Saturn | Mars | Mercury |
| 10 | Pisces | Jupiter | Jupiter | Mars |
| 11 | Aries | Mars | Ketu | Mars |
| 12 | Taurus | Venus | Sun | Venus |

Case No. 024/ dmb
Date of birth 27th August 1987 at 04:30 hours in Pune with
Lat. 018:30N Long. 073:48 E

In this Cancer ascendant chart with lord of ascendant Moon is occupied in third house with sign Virgo. Moon is under aspect of Rahu and is afflicted with Ketu. Second house with sign Leo is occupied by Sun which is lord of second house conjoined with Mercury which is lord of twelfth and third house, Venus which is lord of eleventh and fourth house and Mars which is lord of fifth house and tenth house. As in this cusp lord of twelfth house and lord of fifth house are conjoined it is noticed that even when Sun is placed in own sign because of twelfth house lord associated with lord of fifth house the problems associated with pregnancy occurs. Also, fifth house is occupied by Saturn which is lord of seventh house and eighth house afflicted with Uranus in sign Scorpio. Further lord of sixth house and ninth house is placed in tenth house with sign Aries. Sixth house with sign Sagittarius is occupied by Neptune. Saturn afflicted with Uranus aspect Sun and lord of fifth house Mars indicates acute ailments occurduring the first and second trimester of pregnancy. Moon which is afflicted with Ketu indicates sudden swing in hypertension during pregnancy also as Jupiter lord of sixth house is in quincunx with Saturn and Moon indicates stress disorder during pregnancy with possibility of undergrowth of fetus.

When the native approached doctor as instructed was examined and the cause of stress was her increased blood pressure; it was reported by doctor as high as 180/110 mm of mercury. Probable reasons were not found and were said as chronic hypertension. Accordingly, treatment was administered. In this case it was notable that even when Uranus occupies fifth house with malefic Saturn negative effect was limited to hypertension only. As such native and unborn baby were in perfect health except hypertension.

According to KP system of prediction it can be noticed that there will be safe delivery of child and both mother and child will be healthy. Star lord of ascendant Saturn placed in fifth house aspect Venus which is star lord of sixth cusp and Saturn in quincunx with Rahu which is occupied in ninth house and is also star lord of twelfth house. Sub lord of ascendant Rahu is also placed in quincunx with Venus which is sub lord of sixth house and under aspect of Ketu which is sub lord of twelfth cusp. Sub lord of eighth cusp Jupiter is placed in tenth house. This indicates functional problems during first trimester of pregnancy especially related to metabolism. Though hypertension during pregnancy is likely to cause serious problems related to labor the native did not experience any of such kind.

Planetary Longitudes and disposition is tabled herewith.

| Planet | Zodiac | Degrees | Lord of Zodiac | Star Lord | Sub Lord |
|---|---|---|---|---|---|
| Sun | Leo | 039:29:04 | Sun | Ketu | Saturn |
| Moon | Virgo | 067:02:26 | Mercury | Sun | Ketu |
| Mars | Leo | 038:56:40 | Sun | Ketu | Jupiter |
| Mercury | Leo | 046:02:11 | Sun | Venus | Sun |
| Jupiter | Aries | 275:57:36 | Mars | Ketu | Rahu |
| Venus | Leo | 040:29:52 | Sun | Ketu | Saturn |
| Saturn | Scorpio | 140:53:40 | Mars | Mercury | Venus |
| Rahu | Pisces | 250:12:33 | Jupiter | Saturn | Venus |
| Ketu | Virgo | 070:12:33 | Mercury | Moon | Moon |
| Uranus | Scorpio | 140:02:47 | Mars | Mercury | Saturn |
| Neptune | Sagittarius | 191:40:03 | Jupiter | Ketu | Mercury |

In this table worth noting is that Saturn and Uranus are perfectly conjoined in Scorpio placed in fifth house is likely to cause serious uterine infections and obstructive diseases but as we observe here Jupiter placed in tenth house with sign Aries and Sun occupied in second house with sign Leo provides enough strength to fight with structural abnormalities or infections and as such native never had suffered any obstructive or infectious disorders. Whereas the Mars which rules the flow of blood is conjoined with Sun causes problems related to blood flow which leads to hypertension.

KP House Divisions and Lords of Cusp

| Cusp | Zodiac | Lord of Zodiac | Star Lord | Sub Lord |
|---|---|---|---|---|
| 01 | Cancer | Moon | Saturn | Rahu |
| 02 | Leo | Sun | Ketu | Saturn |
| 03 | Virgo | Mercury | Moon | Moon |
| 04 | Libra | Venus | Rahu | Saturn |
| 05 | Scorpio | Mars | Saturn | Rahu |
| 06 | Sagittarius | Jupiter | Venus | Venus |

| Cusp | Zodiac | Lord of Zodiac | Star Lord | Sub Lord |
|---|---|---|---|---|
| 07 | Capricorn | Saturn | Moon | Rahu |
| 08 | Aquarius | Saturn | Rahu | Jupiter |
| 09 | Pisces | Jupiter | Saturn | Venus |
| 10 | Aries | Mars | Ketu | Mercury |
| 11 | Taurus | Venus | Moon | Jupiter |
| 12 | Gemini | Mercury | Rahu | Ketu |

Case No. 026/nsp

Date of birth 28th March 1989 at 10:50 hours in Guhagar Ratnagiri with Lat. 017:30 N Long. 073:18 E

This chart is also typical representing the pregnancy complications with birth of spastic child. Taurus ascendant chart with lord of ascendant placed in eleventh house conjoined with Sun, lord of fourth house and Mercury lord of fifth house, indicating probable pregnancy complications. Jupiter lord of eighth house and eleventh house is occupied in ascendant afflicted with Mars which is lord of seventh and twelfth house indicates blood related and blood pressure related disorders. Fourth house is occupied by Ketu aspect the tenth house occupied by Rahu with sign Aquarius. Moon, lord of third house is occupied in seventh house with sign Scorpio. Saturn which is lord of ninth house and tenth house is placed in eighth house afflicted with Uranus and Neptune indicates complications in later trimester of pregnancy. Lord of fifth house Mercury is placed in eleventh house conjoined with Sun and Venus which is lord of sixth house indicating abnormalities in either growth of fetus or native's health. As a rule, when lord of fifth house conjoins lord of sixth house it is noticed that neurological abnormalities developed in fetus. Also, as lord of twelfth house Mars aspect Moon the native is likely to suffer from some mysterious diseases during pregnancy which even if recovered lays an impact of fetus. It is observed in this case that after third USG also there was no anomalies seen in fetus and expected normal delivery it is only when in last i.e. thirty-seventh week of pregnancy when native was unable to feel natural pain was required to get hospitalized and after induced pain delivered a baby appearing to be healthy initially. After only few months it was noticed by doctors that the child is spastic having cerebral palsy. Native did not suffer from any abnormalities. This is in fact very much painful for parents to accept their child is spastic. It was studied in detail, but no connecting reason could be established by doctors causing this neurological congenital problem.

According to KP system of prediction also it was confirmed that the native will deliver neurologically affected child. Star lord of ascendant Mars is occupied in first house conjoined with Jupiter which is star lord of sixth house and sub lord of sixth and twelfth house. Also sub lord of ascendant is also Mars is in quincunx with Saturn occupied in eighth house. Mars is also conjoined with sub lord of sixth and twelfth house Jupiter and is placed in quadrant with Rahu which is sub lord of eighth house. This indicates though pregnancy and delivery will be normal, but the newborn will be having some congenital problems.

Planetary Longitudes and disposition is tabled bellow.

| Planet | Zodiac | Degrees | Lord of Zodiac | Star Lord | Sub Lord |
|---|---|---|---|---|---|
| Sun | Pisces | 313:47:59 | Jupiter | Saturn | Rahu |
| Moon | Scorpio | 197:49:15 | Mars | Mercury | Mercury |
| Mars | Taurus | 016:35:25 | Venus | Moon | Saturn |
| Mercury | Pisces | 311:49:28 | Jupiter | Saturn | Mercury |
| Jupiter | Taurus | 009:04:01 | Venus | Sun | Venus |
| Venus | Pisces | 311:49:28 | Jupiter | Saturn | Moon |
| Saturn | Sagittarius | 229:40:45 | Jupiter | Venus | Rahu |
| Rahu | Aquarius | 279:30:38 | Saturn | Rahu | Jupiter |
| Ketu | Leo | 099:30:38 | Sun | Ketu | Saturn |
| Uranus | Sagittarius | 221:33:42 | Jupiter | Ketu | Mercury |
| Neptune | Sagittarius | 228:35:54 | Jupiter | Venus | Rahu |

The native was required to be hospitalized on June 10th, 2015 as 37th week was about to over and doctor decided for induced pain. As it was also fruitless doctor decided to go for cesarean surgery for delivery and operated on 12th June 2015 with successful delivery and safe mother and child. This occurred in Venus mahadasha and when Venus antardasha with Jupiter pratiantardasha was just started. This is very typical to note that even though there was no sign of any disorders functional or structural the newborn child was spastic.

The KP House divisions and lords of cusp tabled on next page.

## KP House Divisions and Lords of Cusp

| Cusp | Zodiac | Lord of Zodiac | Star Lord | Sub Lord |
|------|--------|----------------|-----------|----------|
| 01 | Taurus | Venus | Mars | Mars |
| 02 | Gemini | Mercury | Rahu | Mars |
| 03 | Cancer | Moon | Saturn | Rahu |
| 04 | Leo | Sun | Venus | Venus |
| 05 | Virgo | Mercury | Moon | Saturn |
| 06 | Libra | Venus | Jupiter | Jupiter |
| 07 | Scorpio | Mars | Mercury | Mars |
| 08 | Sagittarius | Jupiter | Venus | Rahu |
| 09 | Capricorn | Saturn | Moon | Jupiter |
| 10 | Aquarius | Saturn | Rahu | Mercury |
| 11 | Pisces | Jupiter | Saturn | Jupiter |
| 12 | Aries | Mars | Venus | Jupiter |

Case No. 027/amb
Date of Birth 11th April 1979 at 12:10 hours in Pune
Lat. 018:30 N Long 073:47 E

Native with Gemini ascendant and lord of first house placed in tenth house conjoined with Sun and lord of sixth house Mars aspect Moon which is lord of second house developed pregnancy diabetes and was required to be hospitalized before even thirtieth week was not completed. Also, lord of fifth cusp Venus is placed in ninth cusp afflicted with Ketu and under aspect of Saturn lord of eighth cusp and ninth cusp indicates obstructive or structural disorders also fifth house is under aspect of Saturn indicating serious complications during pregnancy. Further it is also noticed that Moon which rules the function of endocrine and exocrine glands in body is hemmed in between Saturn and Uranus causing malfunctioning of beta cells in pancreas that causes free sugar in blood. This also has created glycosuria. Also, as Uranus occupies fifth house indicates mysterious diseases associated with pregnancy. In this chart it also can be noticed that the Sun which gives strength for safe and healthy delivery with healthy mother and baby is placed in tenth house afflicted with Mars which is lord of sixth house and in quincunx with Saturn occupied in third house with sign Leo that causes difficult and painful delivery. This is also classical case to study effect of Neptune placed in sixth house indicates serious disorder during pregnancy.

Jupiter which is lord of seventh house and tenth house is placed in second house with sign Cancer and as such protects the unborn baby. As Saturn occupied in third house afflicted with Rahu aspect Venus placed in ninth house which rules the functions of pancreas and as such causes Diabetes during pregnancy.

When in month of March 2004 the native started uneasy feeling with huge loss of energy and sudden fatigue was taken to doctor who advised immediate admission. Then after thorough examination and tests it was confirmed that the native had a hyperglycemia and pregnancy may be endangered as it was Type ii diabetes so also bladder found infected and the infant was at risk. it is therefore doctor advised premature pregnancy termination in the 34th week of pregnancy. The infant was having good health and no risk after birth except underweight.

According to KP system also it can be observed that the star lord of ascendant Jupiter is occupied in second house aspect Mercury which is star lord of sixth house. Also Jupiter is placed in Cancer lord of which is Moon which is also star lord of eighth cusp and under aspect of Mars which is star lord of twelfth cusp. Further sub lord of ascendant Mercury is occupied in tenth house and in quincunx with Rahu placed in third house which is sub lord of sixth and twelfth house indicating onset of complications in period of Rahu Dasha. Also sub lord of sixth cusp Venus is occupied in ninth cusp under aspect of Rahu indicates Venus related i.e. diabetes related problems. In this case as ascendant, sixth cusp, eighth cusp, and twelfth cusp are well connected the disease was expected to occur in the Dasha of lords of sixth house. The native was required to be hospitalized in month of March 2004 when mahadasha of Rahu, antardasha of Mercury and pratiantardasha of Rahu was in progress. Where Rahu is sub lord of sixth cusp and Mercury is star lord of sixth cusp.

It is noticeable here that during first trimester of pregnancy there was not any complications or expected complications which started only after pratiantardasha of Rahu was started and still the health of fetus was fine as against doctor was afraid of.

## Planetary Longitudes and Disposition

| Planet | Zodiac | Degrees | Lord of Zodiac | Star Lord | Sub Lord |
|---|---|---|---|---|---|
| Sun | Pisces | 297:13:20 | Jupiter | Mercury | Jupiter |
| Moon | Virgo | 102:32:28 | Mercury | Moon | Rahu |
| Mars | Pisces | 279:43:25 | Jupiter | Saturn | Venus |
| Mercury | Pisces | 272:52:46 | Jupiter | Jupiter | Rahu |
| Jupiter | Cancer | 035:51:15 | Moon | Saturn | Mercury |
| Venus | Aquarius | 262:08:46 | Saturn | Jupiter | Saturn |
| Saturn | Leo | 082:20:57 | Sun | Venus | Venus |
| Rahu | Leo | 074:11:37 | Sun | Venus | Saturn |
| Ketu | Aquarius | 254:11:37 | Saturn | Jupiter | Saturn |
| Uranus | Libra | 146:34:06 | Venus | Jupiter | Venus |
| Neptune | Scorpio | 176:50:00 | Mars | Mercury | Jupiter |

## KP House Divisions and Lords of cusp

| Cusp | Zodiac | Lord of Zodiac | Star Lord | Sub Lord |
|---|---|---|---|---|
| 01 | Gemini | Mercury | Jupiter | Mercury |
| 02 | Cancer | Moon | Mercury | Venus |
| 03 | Leo | Sun | Venus | Rahu |
| 04 | Virgo | Mercury | Moon | Ketu |
| 05 | Libra | Venus | Jupiter | Saturn |
| 06 | Scorpio | Mars | Mercury | Rahu |
| 07 | Sagittarius | Jupiter | Venus | Mercury |
| 08 | Capricorn | Saturn | Moon | Venus |
| 09 | Aquarius | Saturn | Rahu | Moon |
| 10 | Pisces | Jupiter | Mercury | Venus |
| 11 | Aries | Mars | Venus | Saturn |
| 12 | Taurus | Venus | Mars | Rahu |

Case No. 028/bpm

Date of Birth 27th April 1984 at 11:29 hours in Sindkheda with Lat. 021:17 N Long. 074:04 E

In this chart with Cancer ascendant lord of ascendant Moon is placed in eighth cusp with sign Aquarius in quadrant with Rahu and under aspect of Mars occupied in fifth house indicating functional disorders of hormones and exocrine glands. Sun which is lord of second house is occupied in tenth cusp conjoined with Venus and Mercury which is lord of twelfth house and under aspect from Saturn placed in fourth house certainly causes functional disorders of uterus or ovaries. Also, as lord of ascendant placed in eighth house and causes hormonal disorders or functional disorders of exocrine or endocrine glands is in quadrant with Uranus placed in fifth house and is known to cause mysterious diseases. Jupiter which extends the protection to fetus is placed in sixth house indicating some structural disorders associated with uterus. Saturn, lord of seventh and eighth house aspect ascendant which indicates some disorders associated with fetus. When the native was asked to consult doctor for second opinion about wellbeing of fetus and again USG was studied it was diagnosed the native is suffering from Macrosomia which is typical condition in which excess amount of insulin secreted and crosses through placenta gives large baby or over grown baby. It was confirmed by USG and native was informed accordingly. The native was required to go for cesarean pregnancy for safe delivery of baby. Even after taking every care the newborn baby found some injury during birth. The native was hospitalized in the month of January 2010 and operated on the same day. This was period of Mercury mahadasha with Ketu antardasha and Venus pratiantardasha was in progress. Where Ketu is star lord of sixth house and Venus is Sub lord of sixth house.

Planetary longitudes and disposition is as given bellow

| Planet | Zodiac | Degrees | Lord of Zodiac | Star Lord | Sub Lord |
|---|---|---|---|---|---|
| Sun | Aries | 283:31:34 | Mars | Venus | Venus |
| Moon | Aquarius | 239:52:38 | Saturn | Jupiter | Moon |
| Mars | Scorpio | 121:46:11 | Mars | Jupiter | Rahu |
| Mercury | Aries | 275:16:57 | Mars | Ketu | Mars |
| Jupiter | Sagittarius | 169:19:04 | Jupiter | Venus | Rahu |
| Venus | Aries | 270:16:16 | Mars | Ketu | Ketu |
| Saturn | Libra | 109:54:27 | Venus | Rahu | Mars |
| Rahu | Taurus | 314:41:23 | Venus | Moon | Jupiter |
| Ketu | Scorpio | 134:41:23 | Mars | Saturn | Rahu |
| Uranus | Scorpio | 139:16:39 | Mars | Mercu | Ketu |
| Neptune | Sagittarius | 157:37:47 | Jupiter | Ketu | Jupiter |

## KP House Divisions and Lords of Cusp

| Planet | Zodiac | Lord of Zodiac | Star lord | Sub Lord |
|--------|--------|----------------|-----------|----------|
| 01 | Cancer | Moon | Jupiter | Rahu |
| 02 | Cancer | Moon | Mercury | Jupiter |
| 03 | Leo | Sun | Venus | Mercury |
| 04 | Virgo | Mercury | Mars | Jupiter |
| 05 | Scorpio | Mars | Jupiter | Mars |
| 06 | Sagittarius | Jupiter | Ketu | Venus |
| 07 | Capricorn | Saturn | Sun | Jupiter |
| 08 | Capricorn | Saturn | Mars | Jupiter |
| 09 | Aquarius | Saturn | Jupiter | Mercury |
| 10 | Pisces | Jupiter | Mercury | Jupiter |
| 11 | Taurus | Venus | Sun | Rahu |
| 12 | Gemini | Mercury | Mars | Ketu |

Case No. 029/asg

Native born on 04th September 1985 at 18:20 hours in Mumbai with
Lat. 019:00 N Long. 072:50 E

This is classic Aquarius ascendant chart with lord of ascendant placed in
ninth house afflicted with Ketu, Saturn aspect Moon placed in third cusp
which is lord of sixth cusp indicates sudden complications in last trimester of
pregnancy.

Sun which is lord of seventh house is placed in his own sign, Leo afflicted
with Mercury which is lord of eighth and fifth house and Mars which is lord
of third and tenth house aspect first house indicating healthy baby but native
may suffer from blood disorder especially functional. Mercury which is lord
of fifth and eighth house denotes the abnormal or delayed delivery. Uranus
placed in tenth house is in quincunx with fifth house and in quincunx with
Moon causes disorders related to blood pressure and associated vertigo. Fifth
house is also under aspect of Neptune placed in eleventh house with sign
Sagittarius indicates chronic hypertension that may be noticed in second
trimester of the pregnancy. Also, Venus placed in sixth cusp denotes likelihood
of diabetes in last trimester. As the Aquarius ascendant with Saturn occupied
in ninth house makes native voracious eater the obesity also may be seen
during pregnancy that becomes the main cause of concern. Even though there
was no family history of hypertension the blood pressure was found as high as

180/100 in 29th week of pregnancy, still the unborn baby and health of native was fine. When consulted the senior experts it was diagnosed as hypertension was result of first pregnancy, absence of physical activity and obesity. The native persistently complained about vertigo and was also having nephritic syndrome. The nephritic syndrome means passing of protein in urine as reported by doctors was probably due to Venus occupied in sixth house with star lord Saturn and sub lord Jupiter.

The childbirth was with induced labor, but the health of native and newborn baby was fine due to timely medication and consultation with senior experts. According to KP system also complications during pregnancy are indicated. Star lord of ascendant Rahu is placed in second house with Moon which is star lord of eighth cusp and under aspect from Saturn placed in ninth house which is star lord of sixth house. Star lord of twelfth house Sun is occupied in seventh house conjoined with Mercury and Mars aspect first house. Sub lord of ascendant Jupiter is occupied in twelfth house and aspect Venus which is sub lord of sixth and twelfth house; Venus is placed in quadrant with Saturn which is sub lord of eighth house. Thus ascendant, sixth house, eighth house, and twelfth house are well connected indicating occurrence of complication during pregnancy. The complaints regarding vertigo and feeling of uneasiness was reported in August 2012 but hospitalization and delivery took place in the month of September 2012, when Moon mahadasha and Saturn antardasha was in progress and Venus pratiantardasha was just started. In this case Saturn is star lord of sixth cusp and Venus is sub lord of sixth cusp.

It is interesting here to note that though Venus occupied in sixth house and it is sub lord of sixth house no diabetic condition was noticed probably due to Venus is under aspect of Jupiter placed in twelfth house. Planetary longitudes and disposition chart

| Planet | Zodiac | Degrees | Lord of Zodiac | Star Lord | Sub Lord |
|---|---|---|---|---|---|
| Sun | Leo | 198:16:21 | Sun | Venus | Rahu |
| Moon | Aries | 075:53:22 | Mars | Venus | Sun |
| Mars | Leo | 182:50:12 | Sun | Ketu | Venus |
| Mercury | Leo | 182:30:08 | Sun | Ketu | Venus |
| Jupiter | Capricorn | 344:47:03 | Saturn | Moon | Jupiter |
| Venus | Cancer | 165:07:57 | Moon | Saturn | Jupiter |
| Saturn | Libra | 269:07:26 | Venus | Jupiter | Sun |
| Rahu | Aries | 078:26:30 | Mars | Venus | Rahu |

| Planet | Zodiac | Degrees | Lord of Zodiac | Star Lord | Sub Lord |
|---|---|---|---|---|---|
| Ketu | Libra | 258:26:30 | Venus | Rahu | Moon |
| Uranus | Scorpio | 290:22:30 | Mars | Mercu | Venus |
| Neptune | Sagittarius | 307:12:35 | Jupiter | Ketu | Rahu |

## KP House Divisions and Lords of Cusp

| Cusp | Zodiac | Lord of Zodiac | Star Lord | Sub Lord |
|---|---|---|---|---|
| 01 | Aquarius | Saturn | Rahu | Jupiter |
| 02 | Pisces | Jupiter | Mercury | Mercury |
| 03 | Aries | Mars | Venus | Rahu |
| 04 | Taurus | Venus | Moon | Saturn |
| 05 | Gemini | Mercury | Rahu | Saturn |
| 06 | Cancer | Moon | Saturn | Venus |
| 07 | Leo | Sun | Ketu | Saturn |
| 08 | Virgo | Mercury | Moon | Saturn |
| 09 | Libra | Venus | Rahu | Mars |
| 10 | Scorpio | Mars | Mercury | Mercury |
| 11 | Sagittarius | Jupiter | Ketu | Mercury |
| 12 | Capricorn | Saturn | Sun | Venus |

Case No. 030/das
Date of birth 01st October 1987 at 06:30 hours. in Kolhapur with
Lat. 015:56 N Long. 075:18 E

This chart with Virgo ascendant and lord of ascendant placed in second house with sign Libra and hemmed in between Mars and Saturn and as such indicates obstructive and inflammatory disorders of uterus. Further lord of twelfth house Sun and lord of eighth house Mars and conjoined with Venus which is lord of second and ninth house denotes complications in uterine function. The lord of fifth house and sixth house Saturn is placed in third house afflicted with Uranus in sign Scorpio indicates acute infection and inflammation of uterus especially during pregnancy. Saturn also aspect fifth house and placed in sign Scorpio indicates complications in pregnancy. The lord of eleventh house Moon which rules the hormonal and exocrine gland function during pregnancy. Moon is afflicted with

Neptune in forth house with sign Sagittarius is placed in quadrant with Mars placed in ascendant

Mars being lord of eighth house occupied in ascendant conjoined with Venus and Sun where Sun is lord of twelfth house and Venus that rules function of reproductive organs indicates functional disorders related with pregnancy. When native approached for seeking guidance for if there is any problem related to astrology or planetary aspect and ill effect and if at all is there solution for the same. It was noticed that the native is likely to suffer from certain inherited blood clotting disorder and may also have been suffering from some type of autoimmune disease. To confirm this native was advised to visit expert doctor and after examination and few blood tests doctor confirmed of having previously existing auto immune disorder related to Rheumatoid Arthritis. The native was the accordingly treated with specific medications. Though the delivery of baby was safe and without complication the native was forced to continue the medications for lifetime. Doctor could avoid somehow the probable chances of abortion. According to KP System star lord of ascendant Moon placed in forth house in quadrant with Rahu which is star lord of sixth house placed in seventh house and Venus which is star lord of eighth and twelfth house. Also sub lord of ascendant Jupiter occupied in eighth house aspect Mercury lord of ascendant and in quincunx with Venus which is sub lord of sixth and eighth house conjoined with Sun which is sub lord of twelfth cusp.

## Planetary longitudes and disposition

| Planet | Zodiac | Degrees | Lord of zodiac | Star Lord | Sub Lord |
| --- | --- | --- | --- | --- | --- |
| Sun | Virgo | 013:38:29 | Mercury | Moon | Rahu |
| Moon | Sagittarius | 111:30:55 | Jupiter | Venus | Jupiter |
| Mars | Virgo | 001:19:57 | Mercury | Sun | Jupiter |
| Mercury | Libra | 038:58:17 | Venus | Jupiter | Rahu |
| Jupiter | Aries | 213:16:24 | Mars | Ketu | Sun |
| Venus | Virgo | 024:05:09 | Mercury | Mars | Mars |
| Saturn | Scorpio | 082:17:11 | Mars | Mercury | Moon |
| Rahu | Pisces | 188:21:01 | Jupiter | Saturn | Venus |
| Ketu | Virgo | 008:21:01 | Mercury | Sun | Venus |
| Uranus | Scorpio | 089:23:56 | Mars | Mercury | Saturn |
| Neptune | Sagittarius | 101:35:46 | Jupiter | Ketu | Mercury |

The native was examined for severe pains in joints and reported persistent nausea tic feeling in month of August 2018 and the autoimmune disease was diagnosed. When Rahu mahadasha and antardasha was in progress with Rahu pratiantardasha.

KP House Divisions and Lords of Cuspis tabled as below.

| Cusp | Zodiac | Lord of Zodiac | Star Lord | Sub Lord |
|---|---|---|---|---|
| 01 | Virgo | Mercury | Moon | Jupiter |
| 02 | Libra | Venus | Rahu | Venus |
| 03 | Scorpio | Mars | Saturn | Jupiter |
| 04 | Sagittarius | Jupiter | Venus | Venus |
| 05 | Capricorn | Saturn | Moon | Jupiter |
| 06 | Aquarius | Saturn | Rahu | Venus |
| 07 | Pisces | Jupiter | Saturn | Jupiter |
| 08 | Aries | Mars | Venus | Venus |
| 09 | Taurus | Venus | Moon | Jupiter |
| 10 | Gemini | Mercury | Rahu | Ketu |
| 11 | Cancer | Moon | Saturn | Jupiter |
| 12 | Leo | Sun | Venus | Sun |

Case No. 031/gkg
Date of birth 18th August 1979 at 11:15 hours. In Pune with
Lat. 018:10 N Long. 073:49 E

In this chart first house with sign Libra is afflicted with Uranus indicating weal constitution and prone for mysterious diseases. The lord of ascendant Venus which is also lord of eighth house is placed in tenth house conjoined with Jupiter which is lord of third and sixth house and Mercury which is lord of twelfth and ninth house i.e. lord of sixth, eighth, twelfth house and ascendant are occupied in tenth house with sign Cancer. Also, tenth house is hemmed in between Saturn and Mars indicates acute problems during pregnancy and may cause threat to life of native and child. Further lord of tenth house Moon and lord of seventh house and second house Mars conjoined together indicating hormonal and endocrine secretions which may cause complications during pregnancy. Fifth house is occupied by Ketu and under aspect of Saturn placed in eleventh house is indicating structural disorders that may cause early termination of pregnancy. The native was asked to contact expert doctor for minor blood spot observed and accordingly when expert doctor examined the native it was diagnosed that the pregnancy was associated with unnoticed uterine adhesions that caused spotting. Also, abdominal pains though minor were due to the uterine adhesions and doctor also admitted exceedingly difficult delivery. The USG reports were denoting healthy fetus and therefore native was advised prematurity termination and as such was operated for cesarean delivery. The native was in ICU for couple of days but soon recovered, while newborn baby was in perfect health. Considering the weak stature of the native doctor advised further rest for couple of months to get fast recovery.

The native was hospitalized in the month of September 2008 and was operated next day. This was period of Dasha lord Saturn with antardasha also of Saturn and pratiantardasha of Mars. Saturn being star lord of sixth house and Mars is sub lord of sixth house. According to KP system we can observe that star lord of ascendant is Rahu placed in eleventh house conjoined with Saturn which is star lord of sixth house and Sun which is star lord of eighth house, this indicates the complications during last trimester of pregnancy. Also, star lord of twelfth house Moon is occupied in ninth cusp afflicted with Mars which is sub lord of sixth house. Sub lord of ascendant Saturn is placed in eleventh house conjoined with Rahu which is sub lord of twelfth cusp. Sub lord of eighth cusp Venus is placed in tenth house hemmed in between Mars which is sub lord of sixth house and Saturn and Rahu which are sub lords of first and twelfth house. thus ascendant, sixth house, eighth house and twelfth house are well connected indicating serious complications during the Dasha period of lords of sixth house. it can be noticed that Jupiter which is occupied in tenth house with sign Cancer caused strength and timely diagnosis with successful delivery and recovery.

The planetary longitudes and disposition chart

| Planet | Zodiac | Degrees | Lord of Zodiac | Star Lord | Sub Lord |
|---|---|---|---|---|---|
| Sun | Leo | 301:07:51 | Sun | Ketu | Venus |
| Moon | Gemini | 251:48:57 | Mercury | Rahu | Saturn |
| Mars | Gemini | 252:48:36 | Mercury | Rahu | Mercury |
| Mercury | Cancer | 282:36:39 | Moon | Saturn | Mars |
| Jupiter | Cancer | 297:31:38 | Moon | Mercury | Jupiter |
| Venus | Cancer | 299:09:52 | Moon | Mercury | Saturn |
| Saturn | Leo | 320:47:18 | Sun | Venus | Jupiter |

| Planet | Zodiac | Degrees | Lord of Zodiac | Star Lord | Sub Lord |
|---|---|---|---|---|---|
| Rahu | Leo | 315:30:55 | Sun | Venus | Venus |
| Ketu | Aquarius | 135:30:55 | Saturn | Rahu | Venus |
| Uranus | Libra | 023:34:27 | Venus | Jupiter | Saturn |
| Neptune | Scorpio | 054:11:34 | Mars | Mercury | Rahu |

KP House Divisions and Lords of Cusp chart

| Cusp | Zodiac | Lord of Zodiac | Star Lord | Sub Lord |
|---|---|---|---|---|
| 01 | Libra | Venus | Rahu | Saturn |
| 02 | Scorpio | Mars | Saturn | Venus |
| 03 | Sagittarius | Jupiter | Ketu | Saturn |
| 04 | Capricorn | Saturn | Moon | Moon |
| 05 | Aquarius | Saturn | Rahu | Saturn |
| 06 | Pisces | Jupiter | Saturn | Mars |
| 07 | Aries | Mars | Ketu | Saturn |
| 08 | Taurus | Venus | Sun | Venus |
| 09 | Gemini | Mercury | Rahu | Jupiter |
| 10 | Cancer | Moon | Saturn | Venus |
| 11 | Leo | Sun | Ketu | Mercury |
| 12 | Virgo | Mercury | Moon | Rahu |

Case No. 032/gab

Date of birth 19th September 1983 at 07:00 hours. In Dhulia with Lat. 020:54 N Long. 074:47 E

This chart with Virgo ascendant occupied with lord of twelfth house Sun and lord of ascendant Mercury is placed twelfth house which indicates acute disorders of nervous system. Also, Saturn which is lord of fifth and sixth house is occupied in second house with sign Libra causes obstructive and inflammatory disorders of uterus. Jupiter which is lord of seventh house and fourth house is occupied in third house with sign Scorpio afflicted with Uranus and Ketu, this indicates developmental problems associated with fetus. Further Moon, lord of eleventh house is occupied in fifth house with sign Capricorn indicating hormonal disorders and functional disorders associated with uterus, also as Moon is under aspect of Mars placed in eleventh house which is lord of eighth and third house conjoined with Venus indicates congenital structural disorders associated with fetus. It is observed with this planetary disposition that native may suffer from functional and structural disorders that may cause ill effect on fetus pregnancy. When native visited doctor in the 32nd week of pregnancy in April 2011 for treatment of severe abdominal pain doctor diagnosed the infection of bladder and then all the necessary tests were conducted, it was found that pelvic inflammation was cause. Accordingly, the native was hospitalized and treated. Unfortunately, doctor could not save the fetus and as such was aborted. This hospitalization was occurred on April 2011 when Jupiter mahadasha was in progress and Saturn antardasha with Rahu pratiantardasha was started.

According to KP system also this can be confirmed. Star lord of ascendant is Moon which is also sub lord of ascendant placed in fifth house under aspect from Mars and Venus indicates infections and inflammations during pregnancy. Further star lord of sixth house Rahu is occupied in ninth house and under aspect of Ketu which is star lord of eighth house and twelfth house causes premature delivery. Sub lord of first house is Moon is placed in fifth house in quadrant with Saturn which is sub lord of sixth and eighth house causes hospitalization and threat to life of native. Sub lord of twelfth cusp is Mercury is occupied in twelfth house and is in quadrant with Rahu and Ketu also indicates hospitalization and threat to the fetus life. It was still unclear that the said infection had caused infection in uterus and death of fetus and still not shown symptoms earlier so as to have treated in time.

Planetary longitudes and Disposition is tabled bellow.

| Planet | Zodiac | Degrees | Lord of Zodiac | Star Lord | Sub Lord |
| --- | --- | --- | --- | --- | --- |
| Sun | Virgo | 001:55:44 | Mercury | Sun | Jupiter |
| Moon | Capricorn | 146:27:59 | Saturn | Mars | Jupiter |
| Mars | Cancer | 329:32:20 | Moon | Mercury | Saturn |
| Mercury | Leo | 355:21:53 | Sun | Venus | Mercury |
| Jupiter | Scorpio | 071:15:20 | Mars | Saturn | Moon |
| Venus | Cancer | 329:47:27 | Moon | Mercury | Saturn |
| Saturn | Libra | 038:45:06 | Venus | Rahu | Jupiter |
| Rahu | Taurus | 266:24:39 | Venus | Mars | Venus |
| Ketu | Scorpio | 086:24:39 | Mars | Mercury | Jupiter |
| Uranus | Scorpio | 071:59:23 | Mars | Saturn | Moon |
| Neptune | Sagittarius | 092:52:09 | Jupiter | Ketu | Venus |

## KP House Divisions and Lords of Cusp

| Cusp | Zodiac | Lord of Zodiac | Star Lord | Sub Lord |
|---|---|---|---|---|
| 01 | Virgo | Mercury | Moon | Moon |
| 02 | Libra | Venus | Rahu | Jupiter |
| 03 | Scorpio | Mars | Sun | Saturn |
| 04 | Sagittarius | Jupiter | Ketu | Saturn |
| 05 | Capricorn | Saturn | Moon | Mars |
| 06 | Aquarius | Saturn | Rahu | Saturn |
| 07 | Pisces | Jupiter | Saturn | Sun |
| 08 | Aries | Mars | Ketu | Saturn |
| 09 | Taurus | Venus | Moon | Moon |
| 10 | Gemini | Mercury | Rahu | Saturn |
| 11 | Cancer | Moon | Saturn | Moon |
| 12 | Leo | Sun | Ketu | Mercury |

Case No. 033/ sjj
Date of birth 19th June 1980 at 05:30 hours. in Akola with
Lat. 020:43 N Long. 077:00 E

This is typical chart with Gemini ascendant and lord of ascendant occupied in first house conjoined with Sun which is lord of third house. Second house is occupied by Rahu in Sign Cancer and lord of Cancer Moon is placed in third house with sign Leo and afflicted with Saturn and Mars and conjoined with Jupiter. Saturn is lord of eighth and ninth house and Mars is lord of sixth and eleventh house. Jupiter is lord of seventh and tenth house. Lord of fifth house Venus is occupied in twelfth house. Fifth house is occupied by Uranus. Sixth house is occupied by Neptune aspect Venus placed in twelfth house. Ketu is placed in eighth house aspect second house. Also, Sun placed in ascendant with Mercury is in quincunx with Ketu, which indicates structural disorders of reproductive organs. Also, Mercury denotes disorders associated with epithelial or lining of uterus. Lord of fifth house Venus placed in twelfth house and under aspect of Saturn indicates uterine disorders and also Neptune aspect Venus from sixth house making it vulnerable to cause diseases related to uterus. In this case Uranus occupied in fifth house which indicated mysterious diseases of uterus.

Lord of seventh house Jupiter placed in third house afflicted with Saturn indicates abnormal growth in uterus during pregnancy; in this cusp lord of eighth house Saturn and lord of sixth house Mars are conjoined and indicate serious structural disorders related to pregnancy. As we have observed lord of fifth house Venus placed in twelfth house is under aspect of lord of eighth house Saturn normally indicates complications which are either congenital or developed as structural disorders during pregnancy that cause obstruction and inflammation.

According to KP system of prediction it can also be confirmed that the structural disorders occurred as congenital abnormalities cause complications during pregnancy. Star lord of ascendant is Mars occupied in third house with star lord of sixth house Jupiter and placed in quadrant with star lord of eighth house Venus indicates obstructive growth in uterus. Further Star lord of twelfth house Sun is occupied in ascendant indicates the early termination of pregnancy. So also Sub lord of ascendant Mercury is placed in ascendant which is also sub lord of eighth house. Sub lord of sixth house Venus is occupied in twelfth house in quadrant with sub lord of twelfth house Moon; this causes complications in endocrine and exocrine secretions in body during pregnancy that may lead to early termination of pregnancy.

The native in fact visited me seeking advice over any ritual if I can suggest for satisfactory delivery of baby and may bless health of native. But when the chart was studied native was advised to approach expert doctor to reexamine the native and if required give early treatment to avoid further complications in the month of October when native visited me. After the doctor confirmed that there was abnormal growth of fetus and may not complete the desired period of pregnancy carried out various tests and native was hospitalized. As doctor diagnosed the native was suffering from congenital disorder and the growth of fetus was indicating growth of some uterine adhesions and also abnormal growth of fetus that may give a birth to physically challenged baby if that survives. Doctor advised early termination of pregnancy to safeguard the mother's health. Of course it was shocking to the native and relatives but there was no option but to terminate the pregnancy.

In the month of October 2008 when the native was hospitalized Moon mahadasha was in progress and antardasha of Venus with pratiantardasha of Jupiter was started. Here Venus and Jupiter are sub lord and star lord of sixth house, respectively.

Planetary Longitudes and disposition are tabled as given bellow.

| Planet | Zodiac | Degrees | Lord of Zodiac | Star Lord | Sub Lord |
|---|---|---|---|---|---|
| Sun | Gemini | 004:16:47 | Mercury | Mars | Venus |
| Moon | Leo | 077:36:33 | Sun | Venus | Mars |
| Mars | Leo | 084:54:41 | Sun | Venus | Mercury |
| Mercury | Gemini | 028:10:58 | Mercury | Jupiter | Venus |
| Jupiter | Leo | 070:40:10 | Sun | Ketu | Saturn |
| Venus | Taurus | 358:28:53 | Venus | Mars | Saturn |
| Saturn | Leo | 087:14:54 | Sun | Sun | Sun |
| Rahu | Cancer | 059:18:50 | Moon | Mercury | Saturn |
| Ketu | Capricorn | 239:18:50 | Saturn | Mars | Saturn |
| Uranus | Libra | 148:36:29 | Venus | Jupiter | Venus |
| Neptune | Scorpio | 177:32:07 | Mars | Mercury | Jupiter |

In this chart Sun is occupied in ascendant and aspect seventh house and still the complications occurred.

## KP House Divisions and Lords of Cusp

| Cusp | Zodiac | Lord of Zodiac | Star Lord | Sub Lord |
|---|---|---|---|---|
| 01 | Gemini | Mercury | Mars | Mercury |
| 02 | Gemini | Mercury | Jupiter | Mercury |
| 03 | Cancer | Moon | Mercury | Venus |
| 04 | Leo | Sun | Venus | Rahu |
| 05 | Virgo | Mercury | Moon | Sun |
| 06 | Libra | Venus | Jupiter | Venus |
| 07 | Sagittarius | Jupiter | Ketu | Venus |
| 08 | Sagittarius | Jupiter | Venus | Mercury |
| 09 | Capricorn | Saturn | Moon | Venus |
| 10 | Aquarius | Saturn | Rahu | Mars |
| 11 | Pisces | Jupiter | Mercury | Moon |
| 12 | Aries | Mars | Sun | Moon |

Case No. 034/skk
Date of birth 28<sup>th</sup> January 1980 at 08:00 hours in Pune with
Lat. 018:30 N Long. 073:48 E

Capricorn ascendant chart with lord of ascendant Saturn placed in ninth house with sign Virgo and ascendant is occupied by Sun which is lord of eighth house conjoined with Mercury which is lord of sixth house indicate weak constitution and frequent physical disorders. Lord of fifth house Venus which is also lord of tenth house is placed in second house with sign Aquarius afflicted with Ketu indicating uterus related diseases and probability of miscarriage in first trimester. Also, Venus is in aspect of Mars, lord of fourth house placed in eighth house conjoined with Jupiter which is lord of twelfth house; and is afflicted with Rahu indicating structural disorders of uterus. Sun which is placed in first house and lord of eighth house is in quincunx with Mars and Rahu and as such indicate thyroid malfunctioning, also causes functional disorders related to uterus and hormones. Moon which rules the function of endocrine and exocrine secretions in body is placed in quadrant with Ketu and also under aspect of Uranus that indicates mysterious diseases and Neptune causes problems related to functions of uterus and ovaries during pregnancy that may lead to complications. Mercury which is lord of sixth house placed in ascendant is also placed in quincunx with Jupiter which is lord of twelfth house indicates congenital problems related to uterus. It is also noticed that lord of ascendant Saturn is placed in quincunx with Ketu occupied in second cusp indicating abnormalities and obstructive disorders may occur during pregnancy. When in month of November 2011 native approached me as first time client seeking advice on sleep disorders and fearful dreams she was experiencing; it was revealed that the problem is associated with either hyper thyroids or may be related to abnormal hypertension I advised her to seek expert doctor's treatment with proper diagnosis. Native visited hospital and was found suffering from chronic hypertension associated with higher TSH level; also diagnosed chronic hypertension with superimposed preeclampsia. Native got hospitalized and received proper treatment in time and revisited me after almost one year with cute healthy baby to show me. According to KP system also it is clear that fifth house, ascendant and Venus and Moon are affected giving rise to such problems. Star lord of ascendant Mars is placed in eighth house conjoined with star lord of sixth house, Jupiter and placed in quincunx with Sun which is star lord of eighth and twelfth cusp. Further sub lord of ascendant Jupiter occupied in eighth house conjoined with Mars and under aspect of Venus which is sub lord of sixth house and in quadrant with Moon which is sub lord of twelfth house, also Venus which is sub lord of sixth cusp is in quincunx with Saturn, sub lord of eighth house. Thus ascendant, sixth house, eighth house, and twelfth house are well connected indicating complications that lead to hospitalization.

## Planetary longitudes and disposition

| planet | Zodiac | Degrees | Lord of Zodiac | Star Lord | Sub lord |
|---|---|---|---|---|---|
| Sun | Capricorn | 013:44:29 | Saturn | Moon | Jupiter |
| Moon | Taurus | 147:30:20 | Venus | Mars | Rahu |
| Mars | Leo | 230:51:15 | Sun | Venus | Jupiter |
| Mercury | Capricorn | 018:23:48 | Saturn | Moon | Mercury |
| Jupiter | Leo | 225:01:06 | Sun | Venus | Venus |
| Venus | Aquarius | 050:57:51 | Saturn | Jupiter | Jupiter |
| Saturn | Virgo | 243:02:12 | Mercury | Sun | Saturn |
| Rahu | Leo | 216:53:07 | Sun | Ketu | Rahu |
| Ketu | Aquarius | 036:53:07 | Saturn | Rahu | Rahu |
| Uranus | Scorpio | 301:31:32 | Mars | Jupiter | Rahu |
| Neptune | Scorpio | 328:14:20 | Mars | Mercury | Saturn |

## KP House Divisions and Lords of Cusp

| Cusp | Zodiac | Lord of Zodiac | Star Lord | Sub Lord |
|---|---|---|---|---|
| 01 | Capricorn | Saturn | Mars | Jupiter |
| 02 | Pisces | Jupiter | Saturn | Saturn |
| 03 | Aries | Mars | Ketu | Jupiter |
| 04 | Taurus | Venus | Sun | Mercury |
| 05 | Gemini | Mercury | Mars | Ketu |
| 06 | Gemini | Mercury | Jupiter | Venus |
| 07 | Cancer | Moon | Mercury | Jupiter |
| 08 | Virgo | Mercury | Sun | Saturn |
| 09 | Libra | Venus | Rahu | Rahu |
| 10 | Scorpio | Mars | Saturn | Mercury |
| 11 | Sagittarius | Jupiter | Ketu | Venus |
| 12 | Sagittarius | Jupiter | Sun | Moon |

Case No. 035/djk
Date of Birth 21<sup>st</sup> March 1983 at 23:30 hours in Chalisgaon with
Lat 020:28 N Long 075:01E

Scorpio ascendant and lord of ascendant Mars which is also lord of sixth house is placed in fifth house conjoined with Sun lord of tenth house and Mercury lord of eighth house indicating serious disorders related to pregnancy. Also, Jupiter, lord of second house and fifth house is placed in first house afflicted with Uranus indicates functional disorders related to uterus and growth of fetus. Second house is occupied by Ketu and Neptune aspect Moon which is lord of ninth house and afflicted with Rahu indicating functional disorders related to hormones and exocrine secretions. Fifth house is occupied by Sun lord of tenth house conjoined with Mercury lord of eighth house and Mars, lord of sixth house indicating complications in pregnancy. Also, lord of twelfth house Venus placed in sixth house under aspect of Saturn placed in twelfth house which is lord of third and fourth house denotes disorders related to pregnancy and functional disorders of endocrine secretions. Venus is also lord of seventh house that rules uterus and ovaries. When native visited for finding out auspicious day for function to be held in eighth month of pregnancy and her birth chart was studied, it was noticed that the native must be passing through some problems and when asked, native replied that, it was routine uneasy feeling and little pains in abdomen associated with one or two blood spots. The native then advised to immediately seek doctor's help as it appears to be serious. Doctor when examined;diagnosed as gestational hypertension and was required to be treated with hospitalization for couple of days.

The delivery then carried was normal with healthy mother and newborn baby.

According to KP system it is noticed that star lord of ascendant Saturn is placed in twelfth cusp aspect, Venus occupied in eighth house which is star lord of sixth house; also star lord of eighth house Rahu is placed in eighth house aspect the Saturn, Rahu is also star lord of twelfth house. Further Rahu as sub lord of ascendant and sixth house is placed in eighth house conjoined with Moon and aspect Mercury, sub lord of eighth house. thus ascendant, sixth house, eighth house, and twelfth house are well connected and indicate hospitalization but also denotes safe delivery with healthy baby. In the month of June, the native was admitted to hospital for hypertension Jupiter mahadasha was in progress and Venus antardasha was continued with Rahu pratiantardasha was started. Venus is Star lord of sixth house and Rahu is sub lord of sixth house.

## Planetary longitudes and Disposition chart

| Planet | Zodiac | Degrees | Lord of Zodiac | Star Lord | Sub Lord |
|---|---|---|---|---|---|
| Sun | Pisces | 126:56:06 | Jupiter | Saturn | Mercury |
| Moon | Gemini | 212:24:00 | Mercury | Mars | Ketu |
| Mars | Pisces | 145:16:16 | Jupiter | Mercury | Rahu |
| Mercury | Pisces | 122:19:10 | Jupiter | Jupiter | Rahu |
| Jupiter | Scorpio | 017:14:37 | Mars | Mercury | Mercury |
| Venus | Aries | 159:13:02 | Mars | Ketu | Jupiter |
| Saturn | Libra | 339:40:36 | Venus | Rahu | Jupiter |
| Rahu | Gemini | 216:01:08 | Mercury | Mars | Moon |
| Ketu | Sagittarius | 036:01:08 | Jupiter | Ketu | Rahu |
| Uranus | Scorpio | 015:28:13 | Mars | Saturn | Jupiter |
| Neptune | Sagittarius | 035:35:04 | Jupiter | Ketu | Rahu |

## KP House Divisions and Lords of Cusp

| Cusp | Zodiac | Lord of Zodiac | Star lord | Sub Lord |
|---|---|---|---|---|
| 01 | Scorpio | Mars | Saturn | Rahu |
| 02 | Sagittarius | Jupiter | Venus | Venus |
| 03 | Capricorn | Saturn | Moon | Jupiter |
| 04 | Aquarius | Saturn | Rahu | Moon |
| 05 | Pisces | Jupiter | Mercury | Venus |
| 06 | Aries | Mars | Venus | Rahu |
| 07 | Taurus | Venus | Moon | Rahu |
| 08 | Gemini | Mercury | Rahu | Mercury |
| 09 | Cancer | Moon | Saturn | Jupiter |
| 10 | Leo | Sun | Venus | Rahu |
| 11 | Virgo | Mercury | Moon | Venus |
| 12 | Libra | Venus | Rahu | Moon |

# Chapter 6

# Cancers of Uterus

The term cancer is used for uncontrolled growth of cells anywhere in body in many ways. Normal cell become cancerous when series of mutation leads the cell to continue grow and divide out of control. They have ability to both invade nearby tissues and spread in distant region of the body. Body often may not recognize the cancer cells and as such our immune system cells called natural killer cells which have job of finding cells that have become abnormal and remove them; cannot remove them. There are many types of cancer cells as there are types of cancers, most are named after tissue they have begun to grow.

We are discussing only cancerous growth related to uterus and breasts here.

1. Cervical cancer occurs when normal cells of cervix grow abnormally and details, we have already discussed before and here we shall examine some examples.

Case No. 036/ jjj
Date of Birth 26<sup>th</sup> July 1971 at 09:26 hours in Kolhapur
Lat. 016:42 N Long. 074:13 E

Leo ascendant chart shows lord of ascendant Sun is placed in twelfth house afflicted with Ketu and lord of tenth and third house Venus, which indicates hormones like TSH and FSH secretion disorders causing inflammation and abnormal growth in uterus. Also, lord of twelfth house Moon is placed in ascendant conjoined with Mercury lord of second and eleventh house; this indicates functional problems of exocrine and endocrine glands. Moon and Mercury are hemmed in between Ketu and Uranus and as such likely to cause mysterious disorders. Lord of fifth house and eighth house Jupiter is placed in fourth house afflicted with Neptune indicating abnormal growth of cells in uterus. Jupiter is also under aspect of Saturn which is lord of sixth house placed in tenth house causes obstructive and inflammatory disorders related to uterus. Further fifth house is placed in quincunx with Saturn occupied in tenth house indicates obstructive inflammatory disorders of uterus. The lord of eighth house Jupiter is also in aspect of Saturn indicates obstructive and abnormal growth in uterus. When the native approached me for seeking advice on frequent quarrels with her husband the birth chart was noticed and asked native about any pain in abdomen the answer was not only yes but native added that she has observed few spots also though there was no menstruation last couple of days. It was shocking to me that why and how one can ignore such important sign of threat to life. I asked the native to urgently visit one of large hospital I knew and get examined. The next day only the native called me up and said doctor had advised few tests to conduct and then treatment can be started. As far as age of the patient was concerned at this young age of 23 it was painful to learn she had onset of tumor. After almost week and half again I received a call from the same native regarding doctors finding and was hospitalized for removal of tumor growth as doctor diagnosed her suffering from cancer of cervix. In fact, it was learned later that doctor carried out hysterectomy with consent from the patient and relatives successfully.

In this case it was evident that when sixth house, fifth house, Sun and Jupiter all are afflicted or under aspect of malefic or conjoined with lords of sixth or eighth house likely to lead the growth of malignant tumor in uterus or cervix. In this case Jupiter being lord of fifth and eighth house occupied in fourth house and under aspect of Saturn, lord of sixth house is the major indication that causes abnormal growth in abdomen or uterus and gives early sign of onset of growth of tumor.

According to KP system also it can be confirmed; as the star lord of ascendant Venus is occupied in twelfth house that indicates hospitalization for serious cause and is under aspect of Mars which is star lord of sixth house confirms the sequence of mutations that may cause cancer. Further, Mercury which is star lord of eighth and twelfth house is occupied in first house with lord of twelfth house Moon indicates weak constitution that may makes native vulnerable to life threatening diseases. So also sub lord of ascendant Saturn which is also sub lord of seventh house is occupied in tenth house and placed in quadrant with Moon which is sub lord of eighth house occupied in ascendant and in quincunx with Mars which is sub lord of sixth and twelfth house causes abnormal growth of cells in body which in future may need hospitalization.

It was worth noting in this case that though native was illiterate and was not aware of the life threats listened immediately and approached doctor as advised and could save her life from further spread of tumor in body. But fortunate because, the native had already two kids and was happy with them.

The chart showing planetary longitudes and disposition is given as under.

| Planet | Zodiac | Degrees | Lord of Zodiac | Star Lord | Sub Lord |
|---|---|---|---|---|---|
| Sun | Cancer | 339:04:17 | Moon | Saturn | Venus |
| Moon | Leo | 022:00:59 | Sun | Venus | Saturn |
| Mars | Capricorn | 177:05:19 | Saturn | Mars | Jupiter |
| Mercury | Leo | 005:55:54 | Sun | Ketu | Rahu |
| Jupiter | Scorpio | 093:08:10 | Mars | Jupiter | Rahu |
| Venus | Cancer | 330:07:03 | Moon | Jupiter | Moon |
| Saturn | Taurus | 280:30:26 | Venus | Moon | Moon |
| Rahu | Capricorn | 171:34:33 | Saturn | Moon | Venus |
| Ketu | Cancer | 351:34:33 | Moon | Mercury | Sun |
| Uranus | Virgo | 046:36:50 | Mercury | Moon | Saturn |
| Neptune | Scorpio | 126:55:13 | Mars | Saturn | Mercury |

## KP House Divisions and Lords of Cusp

| Cusp | Zodiac | Lord of zodiac | Star Lord | Sub Lord |
|---|---|---|---|---|
| 01 | Leo | Sun | Venus | Saturn |
| 02 | Virgo | Mercury | Moon | Sun |
| 03 | Libra | Venus | Jupiter | Saturn |
| 04 | Scorpio | Mars | Mercury | Rahu |
| 05 | Sagittarius | Jupiter | Venus | Saturn |
| 06 | Capricorn | Saturn | Mars | Mars |
| 07 | Aquarius | Saturn | Jupiter | Saturn |
| 08 | Pisces | Jupiter | Mercury | Moon |
| 09 | Aries | Mars | Venus | Saturn |
| 10 | Taurus | Venus | Mars | Rahu |
| 11 | Gemini | Mercury | Jupiter | Mercury |
| 12 | Cancer | Moon | Mercury | Mars |

Case No. 037/sad
Date of Birth 21ˢᵗ October 1964 at 10:58 hours in Mumbai
Lat. 018:57 N Long. 072:49 E

This is classic example of cancer of cervix in young age of about thirty years. Sagittarius ascendant with lord of ascendant Jupiter which is also lord of fourth house occupied in sixth house placed in quadrant with Saturn which is lord of second and third house. This denotes obstructive and inflammatory disorders in uterus and causes structural disorders of genital tract. First house is occupied by Ketu aspect seventh house. Fifth house is occupied by Moon which is lord of eighth house in sign Aries and lord of fifth house Mars is placed in eighth house with sign Cancer indicating sudden abnormal growth in uterus and functional dis orders of ovaries. Lord of fifth house Mars in placed eighth house is also lord of twelfth house and indicates hospitalization and surgery. Also, Mars is hemmed in between Uranus and Rahu indicates weak constitution that causes abnormal and uncontrolled growth in secondary reproductive organs. Further we can see lord of sixth house Venus is placed in ninth house afflicted with Uranus indicates poor immunity that fails the elimination of cancerous cells from body. Lord of ninth house Sun is occupied in eleventh cusp afflicted with Neptune so also Neptune aspect fifth house and as such structural disorders related with fifth house that is uterus. Mercury which is lord of seventh house is also afflicted with Neptune indicates abnormal growth of epithelial lining of genital organs, that means cancerous growth in secondary reproductive organs.

When in June 1994 native suffered from dysfunctional bleeding and was admitted to hospital and examined properly. Then Doctor after several tests diagnosed that the native was suffering from carcinoma of cervix with benign neoplasm of uterus. As such native was advised to undergo surgery for the removal of benign neoplasm as well as cervix and uterus.

According to KP system of prediction also it is observed that star lord of ascendant Ketu placed in first house aspect seventh house; and star lord of sixth house Sun is placed in eleventh house as well as star lord of eighth house Saturn and twelfth house is occupied in third house. Sun and Saturn are placed at 150 degrees apart indicating hospitalization and surgery. Also sub lord of ascendant Sun is occupied in eleventh house afflicted with Neptune and sub lord of sixth house and twelfth house Venus is occupied in ninth house afflicted with Uranus indicating abnormal growth of uterine cells that may lead to cancer. Sub lord of eighth house Saturn is occupied in third house aspect Venus in ninth house indicating mysterious disease that may suddenly occur and likely to damage uterus.

After successful treatment followed by radiation therapy; the native got totally recovered discharged from hospital.

## Planetary Longitudes and Disposition Chart

| planet | zodiac | degrees | Lord of zodiac | Star lord | Sub lord |
|---|---|---|---|---|---|
| Sun | Libra | 304:29:18 | Venus | Mars | Venus |
| Moon | Aries | 124:53:15 | Mars | Ketu | MARS |
| Mars | Cancer | 237:57:28 | Moon | Mercury | Saturn |
| Mercury | Libra | 308:10:01 | Venus | Rahu | Rahu |
| Jupiter | Taurus | 150:38:17 | Venus | Sun | Rahu |
| Venus | Leo | 264:35:03 | Sun | Venus | Mercury |
| Saturn | Aquarius | 065:06:01 | Saturn | Mars | Sun |
| Rahu | Gemini | 182:25:07 | Mercury | Mars | Ketu |
| Ketu | Sagittarius | 002:25:07 | Jupiter | Ketu | Venus |
| Uranus | Leo | 259:53:33 | Sun | Venus | Rahu |
| Neptune | Libra | 323:28:27 | Venus | Jupiter | Saturn |

## KP House Divisions and Lords of Cusp

| Cusp | Zodiac | Lord of Zodiac | Star Lord | Sub Lord |
|---|---|---|---|---|
| 01 | Sagittarius | Jupiter | Ketu | Sun |
| 02 | Capricorn | Saturn | Sun | Saturn |
| 03 | Aquarius | Saturn | Rahu | Rahu |
| 04 | Pisces | Jupiter | Saturn | Moon |
| 05 | Aries | Mars | Ketu | Mercury |
| 06 | Taurus | Venus | Sun | Venus |
| 07 | Gemini | Mercury | Mars | Venus |
| 08 | Cancer | Moon | Saturn | Saturn |
| 09 | Leo | Sun | Ketu | Jupiter |
| 10 | Virgo | Mercury | Moon | Mars |
| 11 | Libra | Venus | Rahu | Saturn |
| 12 | Scorpio | Mars | Saturn | Venus |

Case No. 038/ agc
Date of Birth 27[th]January 1961 at 06:29 hours in New Delhi
Lat. 028:36N Long. 077:12 E

In this chart ascendant is occupied with Sun which is lord of sixth house conjoined with Mercury lord of sixth house and ninth house with sign Capricorn indicates invasion due to HPV(human papilloma Virus) which initiates mitosis and mutagenic changes in body. The lord of ascendant Saturn is occupied in twelfth house conjoined with Jupiter which is lord of twelfth house indicates obstructive and inflammatory diseases. Lord of seventh house Moon which rules the functions of endocrine and exocrine glands is placed in fifth house and is in quincunx with Saturn occupied in twelfth house and in quadrant with Uranus and Rahu placed in eighth house; this debilitated Moon causes functional disorders of ovaries and thyroid gland. Further Mars which is lord of fourth house and eleventh house is occupied in sixth house and under aspect of Saturn from third house, indicates blood or exocrine fluid related disorders. As lord of eighth house Sun occupied in first house is placed in quincunx with Uranus gives poor immunity that is required to fight with abnormal cells and eliminate them from our body.

Venus which is lord of sixth and eleventh house is occupied in ninth house afflicted with Uranus; Venus rules secondary reproductive organs and as such cause's ailments related to uterus and pelvic region. Also, Venus is under aspect from Saturn placed in third house in own sign Aquarius. Native visited doctor for persistent pain in lower belly and when doctor examined after few tests. The doctor diagnosed that native is suffering from Adenomyoces i.e. ectopic growth of endometrial tissues within myometrium. This caused severe pain followed by bleeding. The native was admitted to hospital in the month of June 1994 when mahadasha of Sun was in progress and antardasha of Venus was onset with pratiantardasha of Sun started. Where Sun is star lord of sixth house and Venus is sub lord of sixth house.

According to KP system also we can see that the native was prone to suffer from diseases related to uterus. Star lord of Ascendant is Ketu placed in first house and star lord of sixth house is Sun is placed in eleventh house in quincunx with Saturn which is star lord of eighth and twelfth house. Sub lord of ascendant Sun is occupied in eleventh house and sub lord of sixth house Venus is occupied in ninth house which is also sub lord of twelfth house and under aspect of Saturn which is sub lord of eighth house. Thus ascendant, sixth house, eighth house, and twelfth house are well connected indicating occurrence of disease and hospitalization. The native was discharged from hospital in July 1994.

One thing is evident over here in this birth chart that Ketu placed in first house is found to create some disorders related to pelvic region and Jupiter occupied in sixth house diseases related to abdomen. The lord of first house placed in sixth house generally gives sick personality also and because of negative thoughts constantly arising that yields the diseases.

## Planetary longitudes and Disposition chart

| Planet | Zodiac | Degrees | Lord of Zodiac | Star Lord | Sub Lord |
|---|---|---|---|---|---|
| Sun | Libra | 304:29:18 | Venus | Mars | Venus |
| Moon | Aries | 124:53:15 | Mars | Ketu | Mars |
| Mars | Cancer | 237:57:28 | Moon | Mercury | Saturn |
| Mercury | Libra | 308:10:01 | Venus | Rahu | Rahu |
| Jupiter | Taurus | 150:38:17 | Venus | Sun | Rahu |
| Venus | Leo | 264:35:03 | Sun | Venus | Mercury |
| Saturn | Aquarius | 065:06:01 | Saturn | Mars | Sun |
| Rahu | Gemini | 182:25:07 | Mercury | Mars | Ketu |
| Ketu | Sagittarius | 062:25:07 | Jupiter | Ketu | Venus |
| Uranus | Leo | 259:53:33 | Sun | Venus | Saturn |
| Neptune | Libra | 323:28:27 | Venus | Jupiter | Rahu |

## KP House Divisions and Lords of Cusp

| Cusp | Zodiac | Lord of Zodiac | Star Lord | Sub Lord |
|---|---|---|---|---|
| 01 | Sagittarius | Jupiter | Ketu | Sun |
| 02 | Capricorn | Saturn | Sun | Saturn |
| 03 | Aquarius | Saturn | Rahu | Rahu |
| 04 | Pisces | Jupiter | Saturn | Moon |
| 05 | Aries | Mars | Ketu | Mercury |
| 06 | Taurus | Venus | Sun | Venus |
| 07 | Gemini | Mercury | Mars | Venus |
| 08 | Cancer | Moon | Saturn | Saturn |
| 09 | Leo | Sun | Ketu | Jupiter |
| 10 | Virgo | Mercury | Moon | Mars |
| 11 | Libra | Venus | Rahu | Saturn |
| 12 | Scorpio | Mars | Saturn | Venus |

Case No. 039/gur
Date of Birth 26<sup>th</sup> June 1966 at 05:55 hours in Mumbai
Lat. 019:02 N Long. 072:50 E

This is one more classic case of uterine cancer. Ascendant, is occupied with Sun which is lord of third house conjoined with Jupiter, lord of seventh and tenth house and indicates healthy and good immunity constitution. Moon which rules exocrine and endocrine secretions is occupied in fourth house under aspect of Saturn which is lord of eighth and ninth house, moon is lord of second house and indicate the functional problems of glands and organs that secrets these exocrine and endocrine hormones. Also, fifth house is occupied by Ketu conjoined with Neptune and fifth house is in quincunx with Saturn placed in tenth house which indicates the native is suffering from obstructive and infectious disorders of uterus. Further lord of fifth house Venus is placed in twelfth house conjoined with lord of sixth house Mars which indicates the abnormal growth in uterus causing severe pain during menstruation along with dysfunctional bleeding. Also, Venus rules the secondary reproductive organs and is afflicted with Mars as such there is possibility of pelvic inflammation Disease. Moon that rules the hormonal functions is hemmed in between Uranus and Neptune indicates disturbed hormonal balance. When in the month of native visited me for she was interested in purchasing new flat in Mumbai and whether loan proposal will be processed or not I just casually studied her birth chart and it was revealed that the native may face serious threat to her life in coming months. Also I tried to confirm with KP system in which star lord of ascendant Rahu occupied in eleventh house aspect fifth house and Ketu which is placed in quincunx with Saturn, star lord of sixth house which in its turn occupied in quadrant with Sun, star lord of eighth and twelfth house indicating serious threat to life during Dasha period of Saturn, star lord of sixth house. Further, Sub lord of ascendant occupied in eleventh house is placed in quadrant with Mercury which is sub lord of sixth house and twelfth house; also sub lord of eighth house Jupiter is placed in ascendant with Sun and in quadrant with Saturn. This indicates serious disorders of uterus.

After confirmation I advised the native to first take expert doctor's advice and get thoroughly examined for some ailments in uterus, the spontaneous reply was she had menopause in the year 2013 only but since last few days' blood spots are observed with faint pain in lower belly. But assuming it as normal phenomena she ignored. After consulting doctor and conducting some tests and examination the smear sample was sent for test to confirm whether it is benign or malignant type. After almost week native approached me again and thanking me for vital advice on time as doctor confirmed it uterine fibroid with cancerous growth in cervix. After chemotherapy as advised by doctors the native was operated for hysterectomy. In this case the small spots observed after four years of menopause was serious signal but went unnoticed assuming minor ailment. It is therefore very much necessary to take utmost care of even small signs that occur which may sometimes indicate onset of big disease on its way.

## Planetary longitudes and disposition

| Planet | Zodiac | Degrees | Lord of Zodiac | Star Lord | Sub Lord |
|---|---|---|---|---|---|
| Sun | Capricorn | 013:33:05 | Saturn | Moon | Rahu |
| Moon | Taurus | 142:00:00 | Venus | Moon | Venus |
| Mars | Gemini | 157:20:12 | Mercury | Rahu | Rahu |
| Mercury | Capricorn | 027:29:36 | Saturn | Mars | Jupiter |
| Jupiter | Sagittarius | 356:48:45 | Jupiter | Sun | Sun |
| Venus | Pisces | 060:28:48 | Jupiter | Jupiter | Moon |
| Saturn | Sagittarius | 359:20:26 | Jupiter | Sun | Rahu |
| Rahu | Leo | 224:39:12 | Sun | Venus | Venus |
| Ketu | Aquarius | 044:39:12 | Saturn | Rahu | Ketu |
| Uranus | Leo | 211:09:34 | Sun | Ketu | Venus |
| Neptune | Libra | 271:56:11 | Venus | Rahu | Sun |

## KP House Divisions and Lords of Cusp

| Cusp | Zodiac | Lord of Zodiac | Star Lord | Sub Lord |
|---|---|---|---|---|
| 01 | Capricorn | Saturn | Sun | Rahu |
| 02 | Aquarius | Saturn | Rahu | Jupiter |
| 03 | Pisces | Jupiter | Saturn | Jupiter |
| 04 | Aries | Mars | Venus | Moon |
| 05 | Taurus | Venus | Moon | Rahu |
| 06 | Gemini | Mercury | Mars | Moon |
| 07 | Cancer | Moon | Jupiter | Mars |
| 08 | Leo | Sun | Ketu | Jupiter |
| 09 | Virgo | Mercury | Moon | Saturn |
| 10 | Libra | Venus | Rahu | Venus |
| 11 | Scorpio | Mars | Saturn | Mars |
| 12 | Sagittarius | Jupiter | Ketu | Rahu |

Case No. 040/mss
Date of Birth 24ᵗʰ October 1980 at 11:09 hours in Thane
Lat. 019:11 N Long. 072:58 E

This is Sagittarius ascendant with lord of ascendant Jupiter occupied in tenth house afflicted with Saturn which is lord of second and third house. Ketu placed in second house with sign Capricorn and aspect eighth house with sign Cancer. Further lord of eighth house Moon occupied in fifth house with sign Aries is placed in quincunx with Saturn in tenth house and Uranus from twelfth house; also lord of fifth house is occupied in twelfth house afflicted with Uranus and Neptune in own sign Scorpio. This indicates mysterious and complicated disorders related to uterus. Venus which rules functioning of secondary reproductive organs is occupied in ninth house with sign Leo and hemmed in between Saturn and Rahu indicates malfunctioning or functional disorders of uterus. So also, lord of fifth house Mars is under aspect of Saturn and indicates structural disorders of uterus and likely to cause severe infection or inflammation of uterine wall. Mercury which is lord of seventh house is occupied in eleventh house and placed in quadrant of Rahu indicate structural disorders of lining of genital system and diseases of uterine wall. When in December 2009 native approached for seeking advice on change of her job and frequent irritation in relation with her husband it was noticed that there appears some problem related to uterine health and discussed with native; it was stated by native that her frequent mood swing now has become common and her husband is worried about it also there are some problems like frequent infection in urinary tract with reoccurring pains in lower abdomen which subsides temporarily after taking some antibiotics. It was astonishing to learn that the native never had consulted her doctor after her second delivery since last over five years, and self-medication she was consuming. I advised that this is dangerous as we normally do not know the probable aftereffects of different medicines and even the exact cause of our pains. And accordingly asked her to approach expert doctor for further examination and proper treatment.

After almost couple of months again the native with her husband visited me telling doctor had started her treatment and she was diagnosed with uterine fibroids and was advised surgery for the same which was to be conducted next month and for that she needs admission. Native also told me about the doctor also was suspecting cancerous growth and the smear has already sent for confirmation. After almost one year the husband wife visited again with cheerful face telling me that now they have stopped fighting and treatment was successful. Doctor had removed her uterus and given chemotherapy also.

According to KP system also it is noticed that the complication related to uterus are on cards. Star lord of ascendant Ketu is placed in second house in quadrant with Moon which is star lord of sixth house placed in fifth house in quincunx with Saturn which is str lord of eighth and twelfth house. Also sub lord of ascendant Jupiter occupied in tenth house, sub lord of sixth house Rahu which is also sub lord of twelfth house is occupied in eighth house. Sub lord of eighth house Venus is placed in ninth house, as such Venus, sub lord of eighth house is hemmed in between Rahu and Saturn.

The native approached me in December 2009 and admitted to hospital in the month of January 2010 when mahadasha of Moon was in progress and antardasha of Rahu with pratiantardasha of Moon was started. Where Moon is star lord of sixth house and Rahu is sub lord of sixth house.

Planetary longitudes and disposition are charted out as bellow

| Planet | Zodiac | Degrees | Lord of Zodiac | Star Lord | Sub Lord |
|---|---|---|---|---|---|
| Sun | Libra | 307:23:95 | Venus | Rahu | Rahu |
| Moon | Aries | 122:38:29 | Mars | Ketu | Mercury |
| Mars | Scorpio | 345:01:11 | Mars | Saturn | Jupiter |
| Mercury | Libra | 326:15:02 | Venus | Jupiter | Ketu |
| Jupiter | Virgo | 275:47:00 | Mercury | Sun | Mercury |
| Venus | Leo | 268:59:12 | Sun | Sun | Mars |
| Saturn | Virgo | 280:23:24 | Mercury | Moon | Moon |
| Rahu | Cancer | 232:34:20 | Moon | Mercury | Moon |
| Ketu | Capricorn | 052:34:20 | Saturn | Moon | Venus |
| Uranus | Scorpio | 330:45:57 | Mars | Jupiter | Mars |
| Neptune | Scorpio | 357:04:03 | Mars | Mercury | Jupiter |

It is interesting here to note that star lords of ascendant sixth house, eighth house and twelfth house are well connected but sub lords of ascendant, sixth house, eighth house, and twelfth house are not well connected which may indicate deviation from the underlined rule that lords of cusp first, sixth, eighth and twelfth are required to be connected and only then indicate hospitalization and surgery. Also, Moon being lord of eighth house placed in fifth house indicate frequent mood swing which was not appeared before the onset of the disorder.

KP House Divisions and Lords of House

| Cusp | Zodiac | Lord of Zodiac | Star Lord | Sub Lord |
|------|--------|----------------|-----------|----------|
| 01 | Sagittarius | Jupiter | Ketu | Jupiter |
| 02 | Capricorn | Saturn | Moon | Moon |
| 03 | Aquarius | Saturn | Rahu | Ketu |
| 04 | Pisces | Jupiter | Mercury | Mercury |
| 05 | Aries | Mars | Venus | Mars |
| 06 | Taurus | Venus | Moon | Rahu |
| 07 | Gemini | Mercury | Rahu | Rahu |
| 08 | Cancer | Moon | Saturn | Venus |
| 09 | Leo | Sun | Venus | Venus |
| 10 | Virgo | Mercury | Moon | Mercury |
| 11 | Libra | Venus | Rahu | Sun |
| 12 | Scorpio | Mars | Saturn | Rahu |

Case No. 041/bbp
Date of Birth 14th November 1969 at 09:35 hours. in Mumbai with
Lat. 019:18 N Long. 072:51 E

Sagittarius ascendant chart with lord of first house placed in eleventh house conjoined with Sun, lord of ninth house Mercury lord of seventh and tenth house and Venus which is lord of sixth house and under aspect of Saturn placed in fifth house indicates problems of uterine health. Moon which rules functions of exocrine and endocrine glands in body is placed in ascendant and hemmed in between Neptune and Mars indicates hormonal problems. Further lord of fifth house and twelfth house Mars occupied in second house is under aspect of Saturn indicates structural problems related to secondary reproductive system. As Moon is also lord of eighth house occupied in first house indicates disturbed mental condition or presence of some or other psychosomatic disorder. Uranus placed in tenth house in quincunx with fifth house indicates mysterious disorders of uterus or pelvic region. Also, Mars occupied in second house aspect fifth house indicates serious structural problems related to uterus.

The native with good health came to me in May 2010 for seeking advice on her house for whether it has some Vaastu Doshas or what which she believed after she was persistently facing some or other health issues after she shifted to that house. As usual after observing her horoscope out of curiosity I asked whether she had regular periods and normal hygiene, the reply was shocking she did not have periods since last four months and she believed to be effect of menopause. In fact, according to my reading as it appears in chart was, she must have some serious problems. I asked her to consult doctor for the same and when after examination doctor diagnosed her as rare case of uterine sarcoma which means one type of cancer that spreads into muscles of uterus, the native reported doctor that there was dysfunctional bleeding but to very small extent and went unnoticed; so also pains were considered as because of digestive system problems. The native was admitted for further tests and examination and accordingly treated and then operated for hysterectomy in July 2010.

According to KP system also it can be observed that star lord of ascendant Ketu is placed in ninth house aspect star lord of sixth house Moon placed in first house which is also lord of eighth house; star lord of eighth house Saturn which is also star lord of twelfth house is occupied in fifth house. Further sub lord of ascendant Mars is occupied in second house aspect eighth house, lord of eighth house Moon which is also sub lord of sixth house is occupied in first house. sub lord of eighth house Mercury is placed in eleventh house conjoined with Sun which is sub lord of twelfth house. Thus ascendant, sixth house, eighth house, and twelfth house are well connected indicating the occurrence of the disease cancer and subsequent hospitalization.

Planetary Longitudes and Disposition chart

| Planet | Zodiac | Degrees | Lord of Zodiac | Star Lord | Sub Lord |
| --- | --- | --- | --- | --- | --- |
| Sun | Libra | 328:10:51 | Venus | Jupiter | Venus |
| Moon | Sagittarius | 025:17:20 | Jupiter | Venus | Mercury |
| Mars | Capricorn | 043:20:46 | Saturn | Moon | Rahu |
| Mercury | Libra | 326:54:56 | Venus | Jupiter | Venus |
| Jupiter | Libra | 300:29:01 | Venus | Mars | Mercury |
| Venus | Libra | 310:54:56 | Venus | Rahu | Saturn |
| Saturn | Aries | 130:45:52 | Mars | Ketu | Saturn |
| Rahu | Aquarius | 084:22:51 | Saturn | Jupiter | Mercury |
| Ketu | Leo | 264:22:51 | Sun | Venus | Mercury |
| Uranus | Virgo | 283:45:05 | Mercury | Moon | Rahu |
| Neptune | Scorpio | 334:44:49 | Mars | Saturn | Saturn |

In this birth chart it is evident that major planets that rules growth and energy like Sun, Mercury, Jupiter and Venus are placed in eleventh house and are under aspect of Saturn which normally gives obstructive and inflammatory growth in body.

KP House Divisions and Lords of Cup

| Cusp | Zodiac | Lord of Zodiac | Star Lord | Sub Lord |
|---|---|---|---|---|
| 01 | Sagittarius | Jupiter | Ketu | Mars |
| 02 | Capricorn | Saturn | Sun | Mercury |
| 03 | Aquarius | Saturn | Rahu | Saturn |
| 04 | Pisces | Jupiter | Saturn | Rahu |
| 05 | Aries | Mars | Venus | Venus |
| 06 | Taurus | Venus | Moon | Moon |
| 07 | Gemini | Mercury | Mars | Sun |
| 08 | Cancer | Moon | Saturn | Mercury |
| 09 | Leo | Sun | Ketu | Saturn |
| 10 | Virgo | Mercury | Moon | Jupiter |
| 11 | Libra | Venus | Rahu | Ketu |
| 12 | Scorpio | Mars | Saturn | Sun |

Case No. 042/lvc
Date of Birth 24th July 1979 at 22:30 hours in Raigad
Lat. 018:05 N Long. 073:24 E

Ascendant occupied with sign Pisces and lord of ascendant placed in fifth house with sign Cancer and conjoined with lord of sixth house Sun and lord of fifth house Moon. Lord of eighth house and third house Venus is placed in fourth house indicating infectious diseases of secondary reproductive organs, also as lord of fifth house Moon is conjoined with lord of sixth house Sun which indicates pelvic inflammation diseases that causes obstruction in fallopian tubes. Also, Saturn which is lord of twelfth house and eleventh house is occupied in sixth house afflicted with Rahu indicates serious infection and inflammation of uterine wall. Mercury which is lord of seventh house and fourth house is occupied in fifth house conjoined with lord of sixth house Sun and lord of ascendant Jupiter which indicates growth of tumor in uterus or secondary reproductive organs. Eighth house is occupied by Uranus indicates mysterious diseases of uterus.

The native was suffering from abdominal pain and abnormal discharge since couple of months and when consulted doctor for further examination and tests it was diagnosed as Cancer of cervix and was advised to undergo treatment as instructed by doctors. In the month of August 2009, the native was admitted to hospital for chemotherapy and other treatment procedures, followed by hysterectomy in the month of September 2009.

According to K P system also it can be observed that, star lord of ascendant Saturn is occupied in sixth house with star lord of eighth house Rahu and under aspect of Ketu which is star lord of sixth house and placed in quadrant with Mars which is star lord of twelfth house. Also sub lord of first house Mercury is occupied in fifth house with lord of sixth house and in quincunx with Ketu aspect Saturn which is sub lord of eighth house. Mercury is also hemmed in between Venus which is sub lord of sixth house and Saturn which is sub lord of eighth house and as such ascendant, sixth house, eighth house and twelfth house are well connected and indicate serious threat to life requiring hospitalization and surgery.

The native was hospitalized in August 2009 when Venus mahadasha and Venus antardasha was in progress and Ketu antardasha was just started. Venus is sub lord of sixth house and Ketu is star lord of sixth house.

## Planetary Longitudes and Disposition

| Planet | Zodiac | Degrees | Lord of Zodiac | Star Lord | Sub Lord |
|---|---|---|---|---|---|
| Sun | Cancer | 127:37:54 | Moon | Saturn | Ketu |
| Moon | Cancer | 134:40:43 | Moon | Saturn | Rahu |
| Mars | Taurus | 086:25:15 | Venus | Mars | Jupiter |
| Mercury | Cancer | 139:04:25 | Moon | Mercury | Sun |
| Jupiter | Cancer | 142:10:15 | Moon | Mercury | Sun |
| Venus | Gemini | 118:53:35 | Mercury | Jupiter | Sun |
| Saturn | Leo | 167:59:16 | Sun | Venus | Mars |
| Rahu | Leo | 166:48:55 | Sun | Venus | Moon |
| Ketu | Aquarius | 346:48:55 | Saturn | Rahu | Venus |
| Uranus | Libra | 233:21:05 | Venus | Jupiter | Saturn |
| Neptune | Scorpio | 264:29:55 | Mars | Mercury | Rahu |

KP House Divisions and Lords of Cusp

| Cusp | Zodiac | Lord of Zodiac | Star Lord | Sub Lord |
|------|--------|----------------|-----------|----------|
| 01 | Pisces | Jupiter | Saturn | Mercury |
| 02 | Aries | Mars | Ketu | Mercury |
| 03 | Taurus | Venus | Moon | Mars |
| 04 | Gemini | Mercury | Rahu | Rahu |
| 05 | Cancer | Moon | Jupiter | Rahu |
| 06 | Leo | Sun | Ketu | Venus |
| 07 | Virgo | Mercury | Sun | Mercury |
| 08 | Libra | Venus | Rahu | Saturn |
| 09 | Scorpio | Mars | Saturn | Moon |
| 10 | Sagittarius | Jupiter | Ketu | Rahu |
| 11 | Capricorn | Saturn | Sun | Jupiter |
| 12 | Aquarius | Saturn | Mars | Mercury |

Case No. 043/sak
Date of Birth 08ᵗʰ April 1973 at 19:55 hours. in Ahmednagar
Lat. 019:05 N Long. 074:44 E

The native with Libra ascendant and lord of ascendant occupied in sixth house conjoined with Sun which is lord of eleventh house. This indicates structural disorder of uterine tissue. Second house is occupied by Neptune with sign Scorpio, and lord of second house and seventh house Mars is occupied in fourth house conjoined with Jupiter which is lord of sixth house and third house. Third house is occupied by Rahu which aspect Moon, lord of tenth house and afflicted with ketu; this indicates hormonal disorders and functional disorders of uterine wall and ovaries. Lord of fourth and fifth house Saturn is occupied in eighth house and under aspect of Neptune indicates obstructive and inflammatory disorders of uterus. Mercury, lord of ninth and twelfth house is placed in fifth house and under aspect of Saturn denotes the structural disorders related to uterine wall and ovaries. Further twelfth house is occupied by Uranus which aspect Venus placed in sixth house causes serious infection or inflammation of uterus. Sun, lord of eleventh house occupied in sixth house with Venus gives reduced immunity which leads to poor strength of body to fight with Cancerous growth and as fifth house is under aspect of Saturn placed in eighth house indicates abnormal growth in uterus. The native visited to find out the cause of frequent illness in home with unexpected financial losses that occurred over last few months. When the birth chart was observed it was noticed that, some life threatening ailment is occurring accordingly when asked native replied that since last few days she is persistently facing pains and frequent dysfunctional bleeding and also she was afraid of visiting doctor and was seeking some spiritual remedy for the same. Then her family members especially her husband was informed regarding possibility and need to get medical help urgently. After she visited doctor and got examined with certain tests she was diagnosed with uterine adhesions and sarcoma of uterine wall tissue. After almost one-year treatment with surgery, chemotherapy, followed by Radiation therapy the native got recovered. The native got admitted to hospital in the month of January 2011 when Saturn mahadasha, Saturn antardasha and Rahu pratiantardasha was in progress.

According to KP system also we can see that star lord of sign Capricorn ascendant Rahu is occupied in third house placed in quincunx with Saturn which is star lord of sixth house and aspect Moon which is star lord of eighth house and twelfth house. Also sub lord of ascendant Saturn occupied in eighth house placed in quincunx with Rahu, sub lord of sixth house. further sub lord of eighth house Mars is placed conjoined with Jupiter which is sub lord of twelfth house owned by Saturn. Thus ascendant, sixth house, eighth house and twelfth house are well connected with each other indicate the occurrence of disease and recovery.

## Planetary Longitudes and disposition

| Planet | Zodiac | Degrees | Lord of Zodiac | Star Lord | Sub Lord |
|---|---|---|---|---|---|
| Sun | Pisces | 175:07:35 | Jupiter | Mercury | Rahu |
| Moon | Gemini | 244:20:25 | Mercury | Mars | Venus |
| Mars | Capricorn | 105:32:50 | Saturn | Moon | Jupiter |
| Mercury | Aquarius | 147:33:31 | Saturn | Jupiter | Venus |
| Jupiter | Capricorn | 104:36:14 | Saturn | Moon | Jupiter |
| Venus | Pisces | 174:49:05 | Jupiter | Mercury | Rahu |
| Saturn | Taurus | 232:49:08 | Venus | Moon | Sun |
| Rahu | Sagittarius | 078:35:27 | Jupiter | Venus | Rahu |
| Ketu | Gemini | 258:35:27 | Mercury | Rahu | Moon |
| Uranus | Virgo | 357:39:03 | Mercury | Mars | Jupiter |
| Neptune | Scorpio | 043:42:34 | Mars | Saturn | Rahu |

KP House Divisions and Lords of cusp

| Cusp | Zodiac | Lord of Zodiac | Star Lord | Sub Lord |
|------|--------|----------------|-----------|----------|
| 01 | Libra | Venus | Rahu | Saturn |
| 02 | Scorpio | Mars | Saturn | Moon |
| 03 | Sagittarius | Jupiter | Ketu | Saturn |
| 04 | Capricorn | Saturn | Moon | Rahu |
| 05 | Aquarius | Saturn | Rahu | Mercury |
| 06 | Pisces | Jupiter | Saturn | Rahu |
| 07 | Aries | Mars | Ketu | Mercury |
| 08 | Taurus | Venus | Moon | Mars |
| 09 | Gemini | Mercury | Rahu | Saturn |
| 10 | Cancer | Moon | Saturn | Moon |
| 11 | Leo | Sun | Venus | Venus |
| 12 | Virgo | Mercury | Moon | Jupiter |

Case No. 044/snd
Date of Birth 12ᵗʰ July 1981 at 14:05 hours in Nasik
Lat. 020:00N Long. 073:48 E

With Libra ascendant this chart shows typical placement of planet as lord of fifth house and fourth house Saturn occupied in twelfth cusp conjoined with lord of sixth house and third house Jupiter indicating post-delivery accumulation of blood in uterus causing obstructive and inflammatory disorder. Also Moon which rules function of exocrine and endocrine glands and ovaries is placed in second house afflicted by Uranus and Neptune indicating mysterious and serious diseases of uterus. Moon is also lord of tenth house that rules nerve supply to reproductive system which is expected to be affected. Lord of seventh house Aries is placed in ninth house conjoined with Sun which is lord of eleventh house and Mercury, lord of twelfth and ninth house indicating infection and inflammation of uterine wall. Moon being under aspect of Saturn and placed in quincunx with Mars also causes severe depression and frequent mood swing. Lord of ascendant Venus which is also lord of eighth house is occupied in tenth cusp afflicted with Rahu and under aspect of Ketu causes serious diseases related to secondary reproductive system. Further we also can observe that lord of fifth house Saturn is under aspect of Mars which indicates structural disorders of uterus.

When in month of July 2005 native visited me for getting help for her frequent mood swing and irritating nature, I just observed her birth chart which indicated onset of some disorder related to uterus for which there was no answer from her. Then I told her to consult the expert gynecologist with immediate effect. Doctor after thorough examination and tests diagnosed her as suffering from uterine cancer which was likely to have spread into surrounding lymph nodes. Which was causing cramps in back and cranky mood, but no dysfunctional bleeding was observed. The native initially was treated as outpatient but later in August 2005 the native was hospitalized and was operated for surgical removal of uterus and surrounding tissues.

According to KP system also it can be noticed that star lord of ascendant Rahu is placed in tenth house aspect Ketu in fourth house which is occupied ninety degrees from Moon which is star lord of eighth and twelfth house; also Mercury which is star lord of sixth house is placed in ninth house in quincunx with Ketu. Sub lord of ascendant Venus is occupied in tenth house under aspect of Ketu, sub lord of sixth house which is placed in quincunx with Mercury, sub lord of twelfth house. Also, Jupiter, sub lord of eighth house is occupied in twelfth house and placed in quadrant with Mercury which is sub lord of twelfth house. This indicates serious and mysterious disease related with uterus.

In July 2005 Mercury mahadasha was in progress with Ketu antardasha was in its last phase with pratiantardasha of Mercury.

## Planetary Longitudes and Disposition

| Planet | Zodiac | Degrees | Lord of Zodiac | Star Lord | Sub Lord |
|---|---|---|---|---|---|
| Sun | Gemini | 266:18:22 | Mercury | Jupiter | Ketu |
| Moon | Scorpio | 031:56:29 | Mars | Jupiter | Rahu |
| Mars | Gemini | 242:19:27 | Mercury | Mars | Ketu |
| Mercury | Gemini | 246:00:02 | Mercury | Mars | Moon |
| Jupiter | Virgo | 339:46:04 | Mercury | Sun | Venus |
| Venus | Cancer | 291:36:31 | Moon | Mercury | Sun |
| Saturn | Virgo | 340:32:32 | Mercury | Moon | Mercury |
| Rahu | Cancer | 278:44:06 | Moon | Saturn | Saturn |
| Ketu | Capricorn | 098:44:06 | Saturn | Sun | Venus |
| Uranus | Scorpio | 032:40:47 | Mars | Jupiter | Rahu |
| Neptune | Scorpio | 050:10:30 | Mars | Mercury | Saturn |

KP House Divisions and Lords of Cusp

| Cusp | Zodiac | Lord of Zodiac | Star Lord | Sub Lord |
|---|---|---|---|---|
| 01 | Libra | Venus | Rahu | Venus |
| 02 | Scorpio | Mars | Saturn | Jupiter |
| 03 | Sagittarius | Jupiter | Venus | Venus |
| 04 | Capricorn | Saturn | Moon | Saturn |
| 05 | Aquarius | Saturn | Rahu | Moon |
| 06 | Pisces | Jupiter | Mercury | Ketu |
| 07 | Aries | Mars | Venus | Sun |
| 08 | Taurus | Venus | Moon | Jupiter |
| 09 | Gemini | Mercury | Rahu | Venus |
| 10 | Cancer | Moon | Mercury | Mercury |
| 11 | Leo | Sun | Venus | Rahu |
| 12 | Virgo | Mercury | Moon | Mercury |

Case No. 045/ sng
Date of Birth 05th April 1986 at 01:35 hours in Hingoli/Parbhani
Lat. 019:18 N Long. 076:48 E

This is Sagittarius ascendant chart with lord of ascendant placed in third house with sign Aquarius conjoined with Mercury which is lord of seventh and tenth cusp indicates healthy body with healthy but aggressive mentality. But as ascendant is occupied by Mars which is lord of twelfth house afflicted with Neptune denotes congenital or structural disorders of uterus and Mars is also lord of fifth house indicates disorders related to uterus. Also, fifth house is occupied by Venus, lord of sixth and eleventh house afflicted with Rahu and under aspect of Ketu. Venus when afflicted and as lord of sixth house indicate functional disorders related with uterus and ovaries. As seventh house is under aspect of Mars and Neptune indicate diseases related with pelvic region and further, as lord of eighth house Moon occupied in second house indicates malfunctioning of ovaries and lymph nodes.

Native when visited me for seeking some remedial measures for her sleepless nights and disturbed mentality and as such I was looking at her birth chart and observed that she may have some problems related to abdomen or hormonal disorders and asked her to contact doctor is the psychological affirmations and prayers may not work for her. Doctor diagnosed her as suffering from sub mucosal fibroid associated with severe pelvic inflammation disease. Her complaint was sleepless nights, but she did not tell me about pelvic pain, vomiting, cramping pains in back with frequent urge for urination which doctor revealed. She was asked to get hospitalized for couple of days and accordingly was treated surgically and with medication, got recovered in month of July 2015.

According to K P system star lord of ascendant Sun is occupied in fourth house under aspect of star lord of sixth house Mars and in quincunx with Ketu placed in eleventh house which is star lord of eighth and twelfth house. Also sub lord of ascendant Moon placed in second house in quadrant with Ketu which is sub lord of sixth house and Venus which is sub lord of eighth house and twelfth house. Thus ascendant, sixth house, eighth house, and twelfth house are well connected and indicate the serious disease followed by hospitalization and then discharge after recovery.

## Planetary longitudes and disposition

| Planet | Zodiac | Degrees | Lord of Zodiac | Star Lord | Sub Lord |
|---|---|---|---|---|---|
| Sun | Pisces | 111:05:23 | Jupiter | Mercury | Venus |
| Moon | Capricorn | 059:13:31 | Saturn | Mars | Saturn |
| Mars | Sagittarius | 010:08:30 | Jupiter | Ketu | Saturn |
| Mercury | Aquarius | 085:35:18 | Saturn | Jupiter | Mercury |
| Jupiter | Aquarius | 076:22:47 | Saturn | Rahu | Venus |
| Venus | Aries | 129:24:32 | Mars | Ketu | Saturn |
| Saturn | Scorpio | 345:49:09 | Mars | Saturn | Jupiter |
| Rahu | Aries | 127:11:28 | Mars | Ketu | Rahu |
| Ketu | Libra | 307:11:28 | Venus | Rahu | Rahu |
| Uranus | Scorpio | 358:40:56 | Mars | Mercury | Saturn |
| Neptune | Sagittarius | 012:08:44 | Jupiter | Ketu | Mercury |

## KP House Divisions and Lords of Cusp

| Cusp | Zodiac | Lord of Zodiac | Star Lord | Sub Lord |
|---|---|---|---|---|
| 01 | Sagittarius | Jupiter | Sun | Moon |
| 02 | Aquarius | Saturn | Mars | Ketu |
| 03 | Pisces | Jupiter | Saturn | Ketu |
| 04 | Aries | Mars | Ketu | Saturn |
| 05 | Taurus | Venus | Sun | Ketu |

| Cusp | Zodiac | Lord of Zodiac | Star Lord | Sub Lord |
|------|--------|----------------|-----------|----------|
| 06 | Gemini | Mercury | Mars | Ketu |
| 07 | Gemini | Mercury | Jupiter | Venus |
| 08 | Leo | Sun | Ketu | Venus |
| 09 | Virgo | Mercury | Sun | Ketu |
| 10 | Libra | Venus | Rahu | Jupiter |
| 11 | Scorpio | Mars | Saturn | Mercury |
| 12 | Sagittarius | Jupiter | Ketu | Venus |

Case No. 046/spm
Date of Birth 15<sup>th</sup> July 1983 at 17:46 hours in Thane (West)
Lat. 019:12 N Long. 072:05 E

This is a classic case of how growth of malignant tumor is revealed much earlier by using the Birth chart. Sagittarius ascendant chart and Neptune occupied in ascendant indicates weak constitution that fails to prevent the formation of cancer antibodies and there by repeated series of mutations cells get transformed into cancerous type. Lord of ascendant and fourth house Jupiter is placed in twelfth house afflicted by Ketu. Jupiter is also afflicted by Uranus occupied in twelfth house indicates mysterious diseases that may lead to life threatening diseases. Lord of second and third house Saturn placed in eleventh house aspect fifth house indicates serios obstructive disorders of uterus; Saturn also aspect ascendant indicating poor strength to fight with diseases. Lord of fifth house and one year twelfth house Mars is occupied in seventh house indicate conjoined with lord of ninth house Sun indicates abnormal growth of cells in secondary reproductive organs. Also, lord of seventh house and tenth house Mercury is occupied in eighth house indicates diseases related to secondary reproductive organs. Further lord of eighth house Moon placed in tenth house in quadrant with Mars and Neptune indicates functional disorders of exocrine and endocrine glands in body. It is also observed here that lord sof fourth house Jupiter is hemmed in between Saturn and Neptune indicates structural disorders of lymph nodes or secretary glands. When native approached me for seeking some remedial measures to help her husband to come out of financial crisis I also noticed her birth chart and observed some life threatening diseases and to clarify the doubt just asked her any health issues for which she replied no not at all. Again, after almost one year she visited me asking some remedies for her health issues and when discussed she told me that since last few months she is some skin irritation swelling on breast with persistent pain and my prediction seems proved but to confirm and get her urgent medical help I asked her to visit expert doctor in nearing large hospital. In the month of February 2017 doctor diagnosed her as suffering from breast cancer on one left side and accordingly she was treated and operated surgically. Thereafter again in month of December 2017 she was diagnosed the same on right side. Unfortunately, it was difficult to get recovered fully without surgery; she had undergone surgery for twice with tremendous pains, mental stress and financial setback.

According to K P system also we can confirm this prediction. Star lord of ascendant Ketu is placed in twelfth house in triangle with Moon which is star lord of sixth house. Star lord of eighth house Saturn is occupied in eleventh house, Saturn is also star lord of twelfth house. Saturn is occupied hemmed in between Moon and Ketu which are star lords of sixth house and first house, respectively. Also, sub lord of ascendant and sixth house Rahu is placed in sixth house in quadrant with sub lord of eight house Venus. Sub lord of twelfth cusp Moon is placed in tenth house under aspect of Rahu. This indicates abnormal growth of cells in body which may require hospitalization.

In this case native visited me in May 2015 when she was not having any health issues but birth chart was indicating such disease in the Dasha lord Rahu which occurred when native visited back in February 2017 with serious complaint about pains and itching or irritation and was required to get hospitalized. Thus, the occurrence of the disease in February 2017when Rahu mahadasha and Moon antardasha was in progress with Rahu pratiantardasha was just started. Here Moon is star lord of sixth house and Rahu is sub lord of sixth house. This is worth noticing here that we can predict the onset of life-threatening disease much in advance and can guide native to seek medical help accordingly.

Planetary Longitudes and Disposition chart

| Planet | Zodiac | Degrees | Lord of Zodiac | Star Lord | Sub Lord |
|---|---|---|---|---|---|
| Sun | Gemini | 208:49:54 | Mercury | Jupiter | Sun |
| Moon | Virgo | 278:12:18 | Mercury | Sun | Venus |
| Mars | Gemini | 197:14:45 | Mercury | Rahu | Venus |

| Planet | Zodiac | Degrees | Lord of Zodiac | Star Lord | Sub Lord |
|--------|--------|---------|----------------|-----------|----------|
| Mercury | Cancer | 215:38:12 | Moon | Saturn | Mercury |
| Jupiter | Scorpio | 337:44:00 | Mars | Saturn | Ketu |
| Venus | Leo | 249:43:24 | Sun | Ketu | Saturn |
| Saturn | Libra | 304:15:39 | Venus | Mars | Venus |
| Rahu | Taurus | 179:53:23 | Venus | Mars | Saturn |
| Ketu | Scorpio | 359:53:03 | Mars | Mercury | Saturn |
| Uranus | Scorpio | 341:48:43 | Mars | Saturn | Moon |
| Neptune | Sagittarius | 003:34:00 | Jupiter | Ketu | Sun |

## KP House Divisions and Lords of Cusp

| Cusp | Zodiac | Lord of Zodiac | Star Lord | Sub Lord |
|------|--------|----------------|-----------|----------|
| 01 | Sagittarius | Jupiter | Ketu | Rahu |
| 02 | Capricorn | Saturn | Sun | Venus |
| 03 | Aquarius | Saturn | Rahu | Saturn |
| 04 | Pisces | Jupiter | Saturn | Jupiter |
| 05 | Aries | Mars | Venus | Sun |
| 06 | Taurus | Venus | Moon | Rahu |
| 07 | Gemini | Mercury | Mars | Moon |
| 08 | Cancer | Moon | Saturn | Venus |
| 09 | Leo | Sun | Ketu | Mercury |
| 10 | Virgo | Mercury | Moon | Saturn |
| 11 | Libra | Venus | Rahu | Venus |
| 12 | Scorpio | Mars | Saturn | Moon |

Case No. 047/pas
Date of Birth 21ST March 1971 at 11:00 hours in Pune
Lat. 018:30 N Long. 073:48 E

This is Taurus ascendant chart with lord of first house and sixth house Venus placed in ninth cusp conjoined with Moon, lord of third house and afflicted with Rahu indicate structural disorders related to uterus and inflammatory diseases of pelvic region. Lord of ninth house and tenth house Saturn is occupied in twelfth house and aspect Venus and Moon indicating obstructive and inflammatory disorders of endocrine and exocrine secretary glands. Fifth cusp is occupied by Uranus which aspect Sun, lord of fourth house indicating abnormal growth of cells in uterus and breasts. Mercury which is lord of third house and fifth house is under aspect of Uranus and Mars indicates serious diseases related to uterus and urinary system. Lord of seventh house and twelfth house Mars is occupied in eighth house causes structural disorders of ovaries and lactating glands in breast. Mars is placed in quincunx with Ketu and in quadrant with Uranus indicates complicated disorders of secondary reproductive system and breast. Moon which rules function of exocrine and endocrine glands is occupied in ninth house afflicted with Rahu and under aspect of Saturn causes serious diseases related to ovaries and lymph nodes. Jupiter which rules growth and metabolism is occupied in seventh house afflicted with Neptune indicating abnormal growth of cells in uterus or pelvic region.

The native came for seeking guidance on her sleep disorder and feeling heaviness in chest/breast with fear of some serious disease that may require hospitalization. When convinced her about the consequences and benefit that she might get after visiting doctor she prepared to visit doctor. After various tests and examination doctor diagnosed her as suffering from swelling in lymph nodes and likelihood of breast cancer which was confirmed after mammography. She was under treatment for almost one year and after surgical removal of lump that had developed in her breast, she felt recovered and comfort. In most of the cases it is observed that fear and misunderstanding or inadequate knowledge native hesitate to visit doctor and invite more complications. It is therefore becoming necessary spread awareness especially in micro interior area of towns amongst all females in age group of 18 to 50 years.

According to KP system it can be confirmed that prediction of disease is possible to much accurate extent. Star lord of ascendant Moon is occupied in ninth cusp with Rahu star lord of sixth cusp and Venus star lord of eighth and twelfth cusp. Further Venus which is sub lord of ascendant is occupied in ninth house conjoined with Moon which is sub lord of sixth cusp and Rahu which is sub lord of twelfth cusp. Mars which is sub lord of eighth cusp is placed in eighth house; indicating onset of the disease and subsequent recovery.

The native approached me in October 1997 when Rahu mahadasha was in progress and antardasha of Moon was on its way with pratiantardasha of Rahu. Where Rahu is star lord of Sixth house and Moon is sub lord of sixth house.

## Planetary Longitudes and Disposition

| Planet | Zodiac | Degrees | Lord of Zodiac | Star Lord | Sub Lord |
|---|---|---|---|---|---|
| Sun | Pisces | 308:28:50 | Jupiter | Saturn | Venus |
| Moon | Capricorn | 258:26:13 | Saturn | Moon | Mercury |
| Mars | Sagittarius | 223:02:40 | Jupiter | Ketu | Mercury |
| Mercury | Pisces | 323:41:01 | Jupiter | Mercury | Mars |
| Jupiter | Scorpio | 192:59:55 | Mars | Saturn | Rahu |
| Venus | Capricorn | 268:59:53 | Saturn | Mars | Saturn |
| Saturn | Aries | 355:50:25 | Mars | Venus | Mercury |
| Rahu | Capric | 268:11:50 | Saturn | Mars | Saturn |
| Ketu | Cancer | 088:11:50 | Moon | Mercury | Saturn |
| Uranus | Virgo | 138:29:29 | Mercury | Moon | Mercury |
| Neptune | Scorpio | 189:31:50 | Mars | Saturn | Venus |

## KP House Division and Lords of Cusp

| Cusp | Zodiac | Lord of Zodiac | Star Lord | Sub Lord |
|---|---|---|---|---|
| 01 | Taurus | Venus | Moon | Venus |
| 02 | Gemini | Mercury | Rahu | Sun |
| 03 | Cancer | Moon | Saturn | Mars |
| 04 | Leo | Sun | Ketu | Saturn |
| 05 | Virgo | Mercury | Moon | Jupiter |
| 06 | Libra | Venus | Rahu | Moon |
| 07 | Scorpio | Mars | Mercury | Moon |
| 08 | Sagittarius | Jupiter | Venus | Mars |
| 09 | Capricorn | Saturn | Moon | Rahu |
| 10 | Aquarius | Saturn | Rahu | Saturn |
| 11 | Pisces | Jupiter | Saturn | Rahu |
| 12 | Aries | Mars | Venus | Rahu |

Case • No048/spp
Date of Birth 18th September 1977 at 10:10 hours in Delhi with
Lat. 028:40 N Long. 077:13 E

This is Libra ascendant chart and lord of ascendant occupied in eleventh
house conjoined with lord of twelfth and ninth house Mercury and afflicted

with Saturn which is lord of fourth and fifth cusp indicating diseases related to epithelial lining of uterus and urinary tract. Also ascendant is occupied by Uranus which denotes mysterious and inflammatory disorders of internal organs. Sun which rules general vigor and strength to fight diseases is lord of eleventh house and occupied in twelfth cusp afflicted with Rahu and hemmed in between Saturn and Uranus. This indicates poor immunity and causes obstructions in elimination of cancerous cells in body. Further lord of tenth cusp Moon which rules functioning of exocrine and endocrine glands in body is placed in second house afflicted with Neptune and in quadrant with Saturn indicates malfunctioning of endocrine and exocrine glands that lead to structural disorders of uterus and ovaries. lord of third cusp and sixth cusp Jupiter is occupied in ninth house afflicted with Mars which is lord of second and seventh cusp; this denotes structural disorders related to uterus and ovaries. In this chart Sun, Moon and Venus all are afflicted and debilitated indicating serious disease related with uterus may occur. Native visited me for getting cognitive behavioral therapy to overcome the fear factor and depression but when as usual, investigated her birth chart which revealed as above-mentioned serious disease to occur told her to get advice from her doctor. She immediately replied that she is already undergoing treatment for dysfunctional bleeding and persistent pain in abdomen. Doctor diagnosed her as suffering from hyper prolactenemia ovarian cysts; she was admitted to hospital three month back and was operated for removal of ovaries. Since then she had developed acute fear and dissociative depression disorder. The native being an IT professional got herself diagnosed in time and recovered early.

According to K P system also it can be confirmed; the star lord of ascendant is Jupiter placed in ninth house in Gemini owned by Mercury which is star lord of sixth house. Mars star lord of twelfth house conjoined with Jupiter and placed in quincunx with Moon which is star lord of eighth cusp. Further sub lord of ascendant, sixth house and twelfth house is Saturn placed in eleventh house with sign Leo owned by Sun which is sub lord of eighth house. Thus ascendant, sixth cusp, eighth cusp, and twelfth cusp are well connected showing occurrence and recovery after hospitalization of native.

Native consulted doctor in the month of July 2010 when mahadasha of Mercury was in progress and antardasha of Saturn was just started in pratiantardasha of Mercury. Saturn is sub lord of sixth house and Mercury is star lord of sixth house.

Planetary longitudes and disposition chart is tabled on next page.

## Planetary Longitudes and Disposition chart

| Planet | Zodiac | Degrees | Lord of Zodiac | Star Lord | Sub Lord |
|---|---|---|---|---|---|
| Sun | Virgo | 331:36:45 | Mercury | Sun | Jupiter |
| Moon | Scorpio | 034:11:52 | Mars | Saturn | Saturn |
| Mars | Gemini | 256:44:38 | Mercury | Rahu | Venus |
| Mercury | Leo | 314:23:56 | Sun | Venus | Venus |
| Jupiter | Gemini | 250:31:09 | Mercury | Rahu | Saturn |
| Venus | Leo | 301:04:30 | Sun | Ketu | Venus |
| Saturn | Leo | 301:18:36 | Sun | Ketu | Venus |
| Rahu | Virgo | 352:33:23 | Mercury | Moon | Venus |
| Ketu | Pisces | 172:33:23 | Jupiter | Mercury | Moon |
| Uranus | Libra | 015:48:58 | Venus | Rahu | Venus |
| Neptune | Scorpio | 049:58:35 | Mars | Mercury | Venus |

## KP House Division and Lords of Cusp

| Cusp | Zodiac | Lord of Zodiac | Star Lord | Sub Lord |
|---|---|---|---|---|
| 01 | Libra | Venus | Jupiter | Saturn |
| 02 | Scorpio | Mars | Mercury | Moon |
| 03 | Sagittarius | Jupiter | Venus | Mercury |
| 04 | Capricorn | Saturn | Mars | Saturn |
| 05 | Pisces | Jupiter | Jupiter | Mars |
| 06 | Pisces | Jupiter | Mercury | Saturn |
| 07 | Aries | Mars | Venus | Saturn |
| 08 | Taurus | Venus | Moon | Sun |
| 09 | Gemini | Mercury | Jupiter | Mercury |
| 10 | Cancer | Moon | Mercury | Saturn |
| 11 | Virgo | Mercury | Sun | Rahu |
| 12 | Virgo | Mercury | Mars | Saturn |

Case No. 049/rrb

Date of birth 01st June 1967 at 05:43 hours in Bidar Karnataka with Lat. 017:55 N Long. 077:32 E

This is Taurus ascendant chart with lord of ascendant placed in third house conjoined with Jupiter which is lord of eighth and eleventh house, Venus is also lord of sixth house and this indicates abnormal growth in secondary reproductive organs which in due course may lead to cancer. Also ascendant is occupied by Sun which is lord of fourth house placed under aspect of Saturn occupied in eleventh house which is lord of ninth and tenth house indicates obstructive and inflammatory disorders and poor strength to fight with abnormal growth in body. Further fourth house is occupied by Uranus with sign Leo and denotes muscular atrophy and uncontrolled growth of cells. Fifth house is occupied by Mars which is lord of twelfth house and seventh house and indicates structural disorders of uterus; also, Mars is under aspect of Saturn and indicates obstructive and inflammatory diseases of uterus. Fifth cusp and Mars is hemmed in between Uranus occupied in fourth house and Neptune conjoined with Ketu indicates structural as well as functional disorders of uterine wall and lymph nodes. Moon which is lord of third house is placed in tenth house under aspect of Uranus, that causes hormonal disorders and abnormal growth of lactating cells and swelling of lymph nodes. As lord of eighth cusp Jupiter and lord of first house and sixth house Venus are conjoined in third house indicates the abnormal and life-threatening disease related to uterus and breasts.

The native was suffering from dimpling skin on breast and abnormal discharge from nipples, swelling on breast and surrounding part with redness and acute pain. When doctor examined her and conducted few tests confirmed the occurrence of breasts lumps spread into lymph nodes near collar bones. The native was given chemotherapy and surgical removal of lymph nodes and tumor developed in breast when hospitalized. The native initially got recovered but again the growth of tumor relapsed after four years.

According to KP system star lord of ascendant Moon is placed in tenth house, star lord of sixth house Rahu is occupied twelfth cusp aspectstar lord of eighth cusp and twelfth cusp Ketu occupied in sixth house; Ketu also aspect Moon, star lord of ascendant. Further sub lord of ascendant Jupiter placed in third house aspect sub lord of sixth house and eighth house Saturn, sub lord of twelfth house Mercury occupied in second cusp placed in quadrant with Saturn. Thus ascendant, sixth house, eighth cusp and twelfth house are well connected with each other indicating occurrence of disease, hospitalization in Dasha period of star lord of sixth house.

In this case even though Sun occupied in first house with sign Taurus owned by Venus the growth of cancerous cells is not inhibited and led to hospitalization and surgical removal of the tumor.

The planetary longitudes and disposition are tabled on next page.

## Planetary Longitudes and Disposition

| Planet | Zodiac | Degrees | Lord of Zodiac | Star Lord | Sub Lord |
|---|---|---|---|---|---|
| Sun | Taurus | 016:26:11 | Venus | Moon | Saturn |
| Moon | Aquarius | 296:44:50 | Saturn | Jupiter | Venus |
| Mars | Virgo | 141:47:02 | Mercury | Moon | Venus |
| Mercury | Gemini | 037:00:32 | Mercury | Rahu | Rahu |
| Jupiter | Cancer | 068:02:37 | Moon | Saturn | Ketu |
| Venus | Cancer | 000:36:17 | Moon | Mars | Jupiter |
| Saturn | Pisces | 316:42:11 | Jupiter | Mercury | Mercury |
| Rahu | Aries | 341:55:36 | Mars | Ketu | Mercury |
| Ketu | Libra | 161:55:36 | Venus | Rahu | Saturn |
| Uranus | Leo | 116:52:57 | Sun | Sun | Sun |
| Neptune | Libra | 179:07:15 | Venus | Jupiter | Sun |

## KP House Divisions and Lords of Cusp

| Cusp | Zodiac | Lord of Zodiac | Star Lord | Sub Lord |
|---|---|---|---|---|
| 01 | Taurus | Venus | Moon | Jupiter |
| 02 | Gemini | Mercury | Rahu | Saturn |
| 03 | Cancer | Moon | Saturn | Mercury |
| 04 | Leo | Sun | Ketu | Moon |
| 05 | Virgo | Mercury | Rahu | Mercury |
| 06 | Libra | Venus | Rahu | Saturn |
| 07 | Scorpio | Mars | Saturn | Jupiter |
| 08 | Sagittarius | Jupiter | Ketu | Saturn |
| 09 | Capricorn | Saturn | Sun | Mercury |
| 10 | Aquarius | Saturn | Mars | Venus |
| 11 | Pisces | Jupiter | Saturn | Mercury |
| 12 | Aries | Mars | Ketu | Mercury |

Case No. 050/srg

Date of birth 15<sup>th</sup> May 1982 at 12:15 hours in Balarampur

Lat. 023:07 N Long. 086:13 E

First house is occupied with sign Leo and lord of first house Sun is placed in tenth house conjoined with lord of eleventh and second cusp Mercury indicates healthy body and strength to fight with diseases. Lord of fifth and eighth house Jupiter placed in third house is hemmed in between Saturn and Uranus and as such denotes infectious growth in body. Fifth house is occupied by Ketu conjoined with Neptune indicates inflammation and infection of uterine tissue and pelvic region. Lord of twelfth house Moon is occupied in sixth house, which rules secretions of exocrine and endocrine glands and as such indicates malfunctioning of these secretary glands causing hormonal imbalance. Venus which rules secondary reproductive system and organs is placed in eighth cusp indicating serious disorders related to uterus and ovaries. In 2007 May native approached me to seek some advice on recurring pains in abdomen as she could not get relief from the doctor in her village so also, she did have periods since last few months. When her birth chart was observed it was noticed that there must be some ailment related to uterus and ovaries and accordingly advised to consult one large hospital in Pune. After thorough examination and tests Doctor diagnosed that she is suffering from uterine cancer has developed and spread into part of bladder and even breast. She was asked first to get hospitalized and operated for removal of uterine tumor and ovaries including cervix collar. Then she was given series of chemotherapy followed by radiation. Fortunately, doctor could save her life and breast lump was also eliminated. According to K P system also it can be observed that star lord of ascendant Ketu occupied in fifth house placed in quadrant with Saturn which is star lord of eighth cusp and twelfth cusp. Moon which is star lord of sixth house placed in sixth house with sign Capricorn owned by Saturn. Also sub lord of first house, Jupiter is placed in third cusp in quadrant with Moon which is sub lord of sixth house and in quincunx with Mercury which is sub lord of eighth cusp and Venus which is sub lord of twelfth cusp.

The native approached in the month of June 2007 when Rahu mahadasha was in progress and Moon antardasha with Moon pratiantardasha was started. Moon is star lord and sub lord of sixth cusp.

## Planetary longitudes and Disposition

| Planet | Zodiac | Degrees | Lord of Zodiac | Star Lord | Sub Lord |
| --- | --- | --- | --- | --- | --- |
| Sun | Taurus | 270:30:31 | Venus | Sun | Rahu |
| Moon | Capricorn | 169:55:51 | Saturn | Moon | Ketu |
| Mars | Virgo | 036:50:58 | Mercury | Sun | Mercury |
| Mercury | Taurus | 290:12:42 | Venus | Moon | Ketu |

| Planet | Zodiac | Degrees | Lord of Zodiac | Star Lord | Sub Lord |
|--------|--------|---------|----------------|-----------|----------|
| Jupiter | Libra | 069:29:25 | Venus | Rahu | Jupiter |
| Venus | Pisces | 228:30:22 | Jupiter | Mercury | Mercury |
| Saturn | Virgo | 052:49:31 | Mercury | Moon | Sun |
| Rahu | Gemini | 322:28:18 | Mercury | Jupiter | Saturn |
| Ketu | Sagittarius | 142:28:18 | Jupiter | Venus | Saturn |
| Uranus | Scorpio | 099:22:57 | Mars | Saturn | Venus |
| Neptune | Sagittarius | 122:53:28 | Jupiter | Ketu | Venus |

## KP House Divisions and Lords of Cusp

| Planet | Zodiac | Lord of Zodiac | Star Lord | Sub Lord |
|--------|--------|----------------|-----------|----------|
| 01 | Leo | Sun | Ketu | Jupiter |
| 02 | Virgo | Mercury | Sun | Mercury |
| 03 | Libra | Venus | Rahu | Rahu |
| 04 | Scorpio | Mars | Saturn | Venus |
| 05 | Sagittarius | Jupiter | Ketu | Saturn |
| 06 | Capricorn | Saturn | Moon | Moon |
| 07 | Aquarius | Saturn | Rahu | Jupiter |
| 08 | Pisces | Jupiter | Saturn | Mercury |
| 09 | Aries | Mars | Ketu | Rahu |
| 10 | Taurus | Venus | Sun | Venus |
| 11 | Gemini | Mercury | Rahu | Jupiter |
| 12 | Cancer | Moon | Saturn | Venus |

Case No. 051/snk

Date of Birth 07th December 1980 at 22:00 hours in Aurngabad

Lat. 019:48 N Long. 075:19 E

First house is occupied by Rahu and lord of ascendant Moon is placed in fifth house conjoined with Sun lord of second house and Mercury lord of twelfth and third house and is afflicted with Uranus and Neptune. This indicates functional disorders of ovaries and endocrine glands; also, Uranus denotes mysterious and inflammatory diseases of uterus. Lord of fifth house and tenth house is occupied in sixth house indicating structural disorders of uterus and pelvic region. Ketu is placed in seventh house and lord of seventh and eighth cusp Saturn is occupied in third cusp conjoined with Jupiter which is lord of sixth and ninth house indicating abnormal growth of cells in uterus or pelvic region. Fifth house with Moon are under aspect of Saturn indicates obstructive and infectious disease related with uterus. As the Sun is afflicted with Uranus and Neptune the strength to fight with disease is reduced, so also the Sun rules metabolism and as such the native was also likely to be suffered from vitamin deficiency syndrome.

When native visited me in July 2008 for discussing the fate of her newly started business and to get remedial measures for financial progress I just observed her birth chart and revealed that she also must be suffering from some diseases related to stomach or uterus. After I asked her about, she replied that yes, she is suffering from frequent pain in lower belly and abnormal bleeding, sometimes persistent discomfort in lower abdomen with frequent urination. She ignored all these symptoms appearing since last one month. When she was convinced about the seriousness of the symptoms and advised to see doctor immediately. Doctor diagnosed the sarcoma of uterine wall with adhesions in uterus also there was severe infection, accordingly she was treated for cancer with chemotherapy followed by radiation therapy. She was recovered but doctor advised there may be recurrence of the disease and she should check up with doctors regularly whenever called. Later, she did not follow the advice and after couple of years the tumor relapsed, and she was required to get hospitalized.

According to KP System also it can be observed that the occurrence of disease and hospitalization is predicted. Star lord of ascendant Mercury placed in fifth house, star lord of sixth house Venus occupied in fourth cusp and star lord of eighth house Rahu is placed in ascendant in quadrant with Venus. Star lord of twelfth house Jupiter is placed conjoined with Saturn in third house. Sub lord of ascendant Venus placed in fourth house is also sub lord of eighth house and sub lord of sixth house and twelfth house Jupiter is placed in third house making 30-degree angle with Venus. When native was hospitalized in the month of August 2008 it was Venus mahadasha in progress and Jupiter antardasha was on its way with Venus pratiantardasha just started. One important thing to note here is that even the native was seriously suffering from pain in abdomen she did not prepared her mind to visit doctor rather she ignored it causing aggravation of the disease.

## Planetary Longitudes and Disposition

| Planet | Zodiac | Degrees | Lord of Zodiac | Star Lord | Sub Lord |
|---|---|---|---|---|---|
| Sun | Scorpio | 142:09:10 | Mars | Mercury | Sun |
| Moon | Scorpio | 143:03:28 | Mars | Mercury | Moon |
| Mars | Sagittarius | 168:20:15 | Jupiter | Venus | Rahu |
| Mercury | Scorpio | 129:15:03 | Mars | Saturn | Venus |
| Jupiter | Virgo | 073:22:49 | Mercury | Moon | Rahu |
| Venus | Libra | 113:15:37 | Venus | Jupiter | Saturn |
| Saturn | Virgo | 074:39:17 | Mercury | Moon | Jupiter |
| Rahu | Cancer | 020:13:00 | Moon | Mercury | Venus |
| Ketu | Capricorn | 200:13:00 | Saturn | Moon | Ketu |
| Uranus | Scorpio | 123:28:36 | Mars | Saturn | Saturn |
| Neptune | Scorpio | 148:33:18 | Mars | Mercury | Saturn |

## KP House Divisions and Lords of Cusp

| Cusp | Zodiac | Lord of Zodiac | Star Lord | Sub Lord |
|---|---|---|---|---|
| 01 | Cancer | Moon | Mercury | Venus |
| 02 | Leo | Sun | Venus | Moon |
| 03 | Virgo | Mercury | Moon | Saturn |
| 04 | Libra | Venus | Rahu | Moon |
| 05 | Scorpio | Mars | Mercury | Venus |
| 06 | Sagittarius | Jupiter | Venus | Jupiter |
| 07 | Capricorn | Saturn | Moon | Ketu |
| 08 | Aquarius | Saturn | Rahu | Venus |
| 09 | Pisces | Jupiter | Saturn | Jupiter |
| 10 | Aries | Mars | Venus | Rahu |
| 11 | Taurus | Venus | Moon | Ketu |
| 12 | Gemini | Mercury | Jupiter | Jupiter |

Case No. 052/srb
Date of Birth 10th July 1976 at 15:00 hours in Raigad
Lat. 018:16 N Long. 073:46 E

Libra ascendant chart with lord of first house occupied in tenth cusp afflicted with lord of fourth and fifth cusp Saturn indicates severe obstructive and inflammatory disorders of uterus. First house is occupied by Uranus and Rahu which indicates weak constitution of native. Second cusp is occupied by Neptune which aspect Jupiter, lord of third and sixth house causes uncontrolled and abnormal growth of cell in body, especially in pelvic region. Lord of fourth house and fifth house is Saturn placed in quincunx with fifth house conjoined with Venus which is lord of eighth house and first house indicates obstructive growth in uterus and frequent infections. Lord of sixth house and third house Jupiter occupied in eighth house indicates structural disorders of pelvic region and uterus. Sun, lord of eleventh house and which rules the strength of body to fight with diseases is conjoined with lord of twelfth house Mercury in ninth house indicates poor immunity. Lord of seventh house Mars which is also lord of second house is occupied in eleventh house aspect fifth house and indicates structural and functional disorders related with uterus and ovaries. Thus, it can be observed that there is likelihood of occurring serious diseases related to uterus and secondary reproductive system. When native approached me for seeking cognitive behavioral therapy as she was passing through post-menopausal behavioral problems. When I noticed her birth chart and to understand the current physical and mental status it was revealed that there are also other problems associated with behavioral changes, when asked for she told since last few days she is experiencing sleepless nights and frequent sudden pain in abdomen, also few spots of blood were observed. I first advised her to take doctors opinion and then we can continue the CBT. After examination and tests doctor confirmed of, she is having developed uterine fibroid may be even malignant tumor. She was asked to conduct few further tests and scans and was advised to undergo hysterectomy followed by chemotherapy.

According to K P system also it can be confirmed that native is likely to be a victim of uterine tumor. Star lord of first house is Jupiter occupied in eighth house in quincunx with Rahu which aspect Ketu, star lord of sixth house; also, Jupiter is placed in quadrant with Mars, star lord of eighth and twelfth house. Sub lord of ascendant Venus is occupied in tenth house, Venus is also sub lord of sixth house and in 90 degrees with Jupiter which is sub lord of eighth cusp and 30 degrees from Mercury which is sub lord of twelfth house.

## Planetary Longitudes and Disposition

| Planet | Zodiac | Degrees | Lord of Zodiac | Star Lord | Sub Lord |
|---|---|---|---|---|---|
| Sun | Gemini | 264:42:37 | Mercury | Jupiter | Mercury |
| Moon | Sagittarius | 069:47:33 | Jupiter | Ketu | Saturn |
| Mars | Leo | 308:32:10 | Sun | Ketu | Jupiter |
| Mercury | Gemini | 258:28:01 | Mercury | Venus | Moon |
| Jupiter | Taurus | 210:20:41 | Venus | Sun | Saturn |
| Venus | Cancer | 270:49:35 | Moon | Jupiter | Mars |
| Saturn | Cancer | 280:33:47 | Moon | Saturn | Sun |
| Rahu | Libra | 015:35:43 | Venus | Rahu | Venus |
| Ketu | Aries | 195:35:43 | Mars | Venus | Sun |
| Uranus | Libra | 009:30:10 | Venus | Rahu | Jupiter |
| Neptune | Scorpio | 048:08:30 | Mars | Mercury | Mercury |

## KP House Divisions and Lords of Cusp

| Cusp | Zodiac | Lord of Zodiac | Star Lord | Sub lord |
|---|---|---|---|---|
| 01 | Libra | Venus | Jupiter | Venus |
| 02 | Scorpio | Mars | Mercury | Jupiter |
| 03 | Sagittarius | Jupiter | Sun | Sun |
| 04 | Capricorn | Saturn | Mars | Saturn |
| 05 | Pisces | Jupiter | Jupiter | Mars |
| 06 | Aries | Mars | Ketu | Venus |
| 07 | Aries | Mars | Sun | Moon |
| 08 | Taurus | Venus | Mars | Jupiter |
| 09 | Gemini | Mercury | Jupiter | Venus |
| 10 | Cancer | Moon | Mercury | Saturn |
| 11 | Virgo | Mercury | Sun | Rahu |
| 12 | Libra | Venus | Mars | Mercury |

Case No. 053/ssa

Date of birth 07th December 1980 at 22:00 hours in Aurangabad

Lat. 019:48 N Long. 075:19 E

First house is occupied by Rahu in sign Cancer and lord of ascendant is placed in fifth house conjoined with Sun which is lord of second cusp and Mercury which is lord of third and twelfth cusp afflicted with Uranus which indicates mysterious and infectious diseases and Neptune. Lord of fourth house and eleventh cusp Venus is placed in fourth house in quadrant with Rahu indicates native is likely to suffer from inflammatory diseases related to uterus. Seventh cusp is occupied by Ketu. Moon is afflicted with Uranus and Neptune and under aspect of Saturn indicates structural disorders related to uterine wall or tissues and other secondary reproductive organs. Sun is also afflicted with Uranus and Neptune and denotes reduced immunity and strength to fight with diseases. As Venus which rules functioning of secondary reproductive organs and hemmed in between Saturn and Uranus causes abnormal and uncontrolled growth of thyroid gland and lactating glands of breasts. Jupiter lord of sixth house occupied in third cusp afflicted with Saturn indicate uncontrolled and abnormal growth of cells anywhere in body. Native visited me for seeking some prayer or pooja to be performed for better health of her and her husband; when I had seen birth charts of both her husband was only suffering from dissociative depression disorder which was treated by extending Rational Emotive Therapy and periodic counseling. For her when I observed the birth chart it was noticed that she is passing through tremendous painful condition and when asked she told me that there is heaviness in chest with swelling and persistent watery discharge through nipples. She also complained that after her last pregnancy she is consistently facing infection in urinary tract. As we have seen into her chart discussed above, I advised her to visit expert Gynecologist and consult oncologist to confirm there is no threat of cancer. Due to her age under thirty I felt it is impossible she may have cancer but exactly opposite was the fact. Doctor after examination and necessary tests diagnosed her as case of advanced breast cancer which was spread into her collar bone also needing urgent surgical treatment. She was hospitalized in August 2008 and after surgical removal of her breast she was under treatment for almost year and half. She got recovered in 2009 but again the tumor reappeared in 2014 thereafter was under treatment in various hospitals but doctors could not save her life.

According to K P system also it can be confirmed. Star lord of ascendant Mercury is occupied in fifth cusp, star lord of sixth house Venus is placed in fourth house in quadrant with Venus which is star lord of eighth cusp. Star lord of twelfth cusp is occupied in third house in sign Virgo owned by Mercury. Also sub lord of ascendant and eighth house Venus is placed in forth house and sub lord of sixth house and twelfth house Jupiter occupied in third cusp indicates hospitalization and surgery.

| Planet | Zodiac | Degrees | Lord of Zodiac | Star Lord | Sub Lord |
|---|---|---|---|---|---|
| Sun | Scorpio | 142:09:10 | Mars | Mercury | Sun |
| Moon | Scorpio | 143:03:28 | Mars | Mercury | Moon |
| Mars | Sagittarius | 168:20:15 | Jupiter | Venus | Rahu |
| Mercury | Scorpio | 129:15:03 | Mars | Saturn | Venus |
| Jupiter | Virgo | 073:22:49 | Mercury | Moon | Rahu |
| Venus | Libra | 113:15:37 | Venus | Jupiter | Saturn |
| Saturn | Virgo | 074:39:17 | Mercury | Moon | Jupiter |
| Rahu | Cancer | 020:13:00 | Moon | Mercury | Venus |
| Ketu | Capricorn | 200:13:00 | Saturn | Moon | Ketu |
| Uranus | Scorpio | 123:28:36 | Mars | Saturn | Saturn |
| Neptune | Scorpio | 148:33:18 | Mars | Mercury | Saturn |

## KP House Divisions and Lords of Cusp

| Cusp | Zodiac | Lord of Zodiac | Star Lord | Sub Lord |
|---|---|---|---|---|
| 01 | Cancer | Moon | Mercury | Venus |
| 02 | Leo | Sun | Venus | Moon |
| 03 | Virgo | Mercury | Moon | Saturn |
| 04 | Libra | Venus | Rahu | Moon |
| 05 | Scorpio | Mars | Mercury | Venus |
| 06 | Sagittarius | Jupiter | Venus | Jupiter |
| 07 | Capricorn | Saturn | Moon | Ketu |
| 08 | Aquarius | Saturn | Rahu | Venus |
| 09 | Pisces | Jupiter | Saturn | Jupiter |
| 10 | Aries | Mars | Venus | Rahu |
| 11 | Taurus | Venus | Moon | Ketu |
| 12 | Gemini | Mercury | Jupiter | Jupiter |

Case No. 054/ ssa

Date of birth 21st November 1968 at 04:30 hours in Mumbai

Lat. 019:05 N Long. 072:54 E

This is classic case of post-menopausal complications and disorders related to endocrine glands. Ascendant is occupied by Mercury with sign Libra and lord of ascendant placed in third house. Mercury is hemmed in between Mars,

Uranus in twelfth cusp and Neptune in second cusp indicates functional disorders of sympathetic and para sympathetic nervous system. Venus lord of first house is under aspect of Saturn placed in sixth house and Mars occupied in twelfth house indicates structural and functional disorders of reproductive system. Sun lord of eleventh cusp which rules metabolism and phosphorylation reactions in body that generate energy, is placed afflicted with Neptune indicates poor strength to fight with adverse situations and reduces immunity. Moon which rules functions of exocrine and endocrine glands and functions of involuntary nervous system is afflicted with Neptune gives nervous disorders and functional disorders of endocrine and exocrine glands. Lord of fifth cusp and fourth cusp Saturn is occupied in sixth house afflicted with Rahu indicate serious obstructive and inflammatory diseases of uterus. Lord of seventh and second house Mars is occupied in twelfth house conjoined with lord of sixth cusp Jupiter and afflicted with Uranus and Neptune indicates structural disorders of reproductive system and blood disorders.

The native approached me to find solution for her frequent erratic behavior at home sleepless nights. When her birth chart was studied it was noticed that she must be having some problems related to lumps in breast and /or uterine wall and accordingly advised her to consult expert doctor then this behavioral treatment can be given. After she got examined and got tested by doctor she was diagnosed as suffering from breast tumor and cancerous growth around cervix. She was given treatment followed by surgical removal of breast and after almost one year she came back to me thanking me. According to K P system also it can be observed that star lord of first house Mars is placed in twelfth house under aspect of Saturn which is star lord of sixth house and in triangle with Sun which is star lord of eighth house and twelfth house. Also sub lord of ascendant Venus occupied in third cusp placed in quadrant with Saturn which is sub lord of sixth house and twelfth house placed in sixth house; sub lord of eighth house Jupiter is placed in quadrant with Venus indicates abnormal growth of cells in secondary reproductive system and tissues around. Thus ascendant, sixth house, eighth cusp and twelfth cusp are well connected causing hospitalization and surgery. The native approached me in the month of May 2019 when mahadasha of Sun was in progress and antardasha with pratiantardasha of Saturn was started. Saturn is star lord and sub lord of sixth house.

## Planetary longitudes and disposition

| Planet | Zodiac | Degrees | Lord of Zodiac | Star Lord | Sub Lord |
|---|---|---|---|---|---|
| Sun | Scorpio | 035:16:51 | Mars | Saturn | Saturn |
| Moon | Scorpio | 044:10:05 | Mars | Saturn | Rahu |
| Mars | Virgo | 343:39:53 | Mercury | Moon | Rahu |
| Mercury | Libra | 026:09:34 | Venus | Jupiter | Ketu |
| Jupiter | Virgo | 337:23:20 | Mercury | Sun | Ketu |
| Venus | Sagittarius | 073:52:55 | Jupiter | Venus | Venus |
| Saturn | Pisces | 176:06:09 | Jupiter | Mercury | Rahu |
| Rahu | Pisces | 163:21:53 | Jupiter | Saturn | Rahu |
| Ketu | Virgo | 343:21:53 | Mercury | Moon | Rahu |
| Uranus | Virgo | 339:31:21 | Mercury | Sun | Venus |
| Neptune | Scorpio | 032:55:39 | Mars | Jupiter | Rahu |

## KP House divisions and Lords of Cusp

| Cusp | Zodiac | Lord of Zodiac | Star Lord | Sub Lord |
|---|---|---|---|---|
| 01 | Libra | Venus | Mars | Venus |
| 02 | Scorpio | Mars | Jupiter | Rahu |
| 03 | Sagittarius | Jupiter | Ketu | Venus |
| 04 | Capricorn | Saturn | Sun | Jupiter |
| 05 | Aquarius | Saturn | Mars | Venus |
| 06 | Pisces | Jupiter | Saturn | Saturn |
| 07 | Aries | Mars | Ketu | Venus |
| 08 | Taurus | Venus | Sun | Jupiter |
| 09 | Gemini | Mercury | Mars | Ketu |
| 10 | Cancer | Moon | Jupiter | Rahu |
| 11 | Leo | Sun | Ketu | Moon |
| 12 | Virgo | Mercury | Sun | Saturn |

It can be summarized that we can predict the disease before it occurs and must act accordingly. It is also unfortunately observed that in most of the cases the problems related with uterine health are not at all given timely attention and therefore problems worsen. Awareness to consult doctor for even small problem related with uterine health certainly will help avoiding further complications and even financial losses to our community.

# Chapter 7

# Breast Cancer and Planets

Breast cancer is the most common invasive cancer in women and second leading cause of death in women after lung cancer. according to World Health Organization records there are 13.1 million breast cancer survivors in the world and the chance of woman dying from breast cancer is around 1 in 38 i.e. approximately 2.6% and becomes major cause of death.

Symptoms: the advances in screening and the treatment for breast cancer have improved survival rate dramatically since 1989. Awareness of the symptoms and need for screening are important ways of reducing the risk and furthermore if the probability of occurring breast cancer be predicted in early life then even before symptom occur preventive measures can be taken.

Symptoms: the first symptoms of breast cancer usually appear as an area of thickened tissue in the breast or a lump in the breast or in armpit may be noticed.

Other symptoms include as:
1. Pain in the armpit or breast that does not change with the monthly cycle.
2. Pitting or redness of skin of the breast similar to the surface of an orange.
3. A rash around or on one of the nipples possibly with little pain.
4. Abnormal discharge from nipple sometimes containing blood.
5. A sunken or inverted nipple
6. A change in the size or shape of the breast.
7. Peeling, flaking or scaling of the skin on the breast or nipple.
8. Most breast lumps develop into cancer and according to size of the tumor and whether it has spread to lymph nodes or other parts of body the

approximate stage of the growth can be determined. There are different ways of staging breast cancer; one way is from stage 0-4 with subdivided categories at each numbered stage. Description of the four main stages are any listed below though the specific substage of cancer may also depend upon other specific characteristics of the tumor such as HER2 receptor status.

➤ Stage 0: this is known as ductal carcinoma in situ (DCIS), the cells in this stage are limited to within the duct and have not invaded surrounding tissues.

➤ Stage 1: at this stage the tumor measure up to 2 centimeter across. It has not affected any lymph node or there are small groups of cancer cells in the lymph nodes.

➤ Stage 2: the tumor is 2 centimeters across and it has started to spread to nearby nodes or is 2-5 centimeter across and has not spread to the lymph nodes.

➤ Stage 3: the tumor is 5 centimeter across and it has spread to several lymph nodes or the tumor is larger than 5 centimeter across and has spread to few lymph nodes.

➤ Stage 4: the cancer has spread to distant organs, most often the bones or liver or brain and lungs.

➤ Causes: After puberty woman's breast consists of fat, connective tissue and thousands of lobules which are tiny glands that produce milk for breast feeding. Tiny tubes or ducts carry the milk towards the nipple. Cancer causes the cells to multiply uncontrollably; cells do not die at the usual point of their life cycle. This excessive cell growth causes cancer because the tumor uses nutrients and energy and deprives the cells around it. Breast cancer usually starts in the inner lining of milk ducts or the lobules that produce and supply milk to nipple. Exact cause of breast cancer remains unclear risk factors make it more likely. It is possible to prevent some of these risk factors,

1. Age the risk of breast cancer increases with age at the age of 20 years the chance of developing breast cancer in the next decade when we say 1 in 8 i.e. means around 12% women are likely to develop breast cancer.

2. Obesity or overweight, women with who became overweight after menopause are likely to suffer breast cancer due to increased estrogen level or even high sugar intake.

3.  Alcohol consumption, alcohol consumption plays a definite role in development of breast cancer.
4.  Radiation exposure, undergoing radiation may increase the risk of developing breast cancer.
5.  Hormone treatment, oral contraceptives increases the risk of breast cancer; also, HRT or hormone replacement therapy specifically EPT estrogen progesterone therapy is related to an increased risk of breast cancer.
6.  Ovary malfunctioning, According to American Cancer Society the abnormal functioning or functional disorder of ovaries lead to the development of breast cancer.

To understand this, we can refer to few examples who have suffered from breast cancer as given below.

Case No. 055/svg
Date of Birth 02nd May 1976 at 04:36 hours in Pune with
Lat. 018:30 N Long. 073:48 E

This is classic case of Breast cancer and birth chart shows Pisces falls in ascendant and the lord of Jupiter ascendant occupied in second house with sign Aries. Jupiter is conjoined with Venus which is lord of third and eighth cusp and Sun which is lord of sixth house and afflicted with Ketu, this indicates that the native is having poor strength to fight with adversaries and also due to poor immunity the growth of cancerous cells. The Moon which is lord of fifth house is placed in third house conjoined with Mercury which is lord of seventh and fourth house and is hemmed in between Ketu and Mars, this indicates the functional problems associated with secondary reproductive organs; also lord of ninth house and second house Mars is placed in fourth house which rules blood vessels and functioning of lymph nodes, Mars is placed in quincunx with Neptune occupied in ninth house causes mal functioning of immunity system and lymph nodes. Fifth house is occupied by Saturn which is lord of twelfth cusp and indicates obstructive and inflammatory disorders of uterus. Further Jupiter which rules health and growth of cells in body is placed in quadrant with Saturn and afflicted with Ketu increases the probability of abnormal growth of cells and malfunctioning of immunity system. Also it can be seen that lord of sixth house, lord of eighth house and lord of ascendant are con joined in second house indicates the poor strength to fight with abnormal growth of cells in body also indicate the malfunctioning of exocrine and endocrine gland.

The native approached for seeking some behavioral therapy to drive away the low feeling and persistently depressed mood or even cranky mood often but when the birth chart studied it was noticed that the native is likely to suffer from life threatening disease like cancer. Accordingly, when asked the native replied since last month she was suffering from little consistent pain on one side in breast and reported something like watery is oozing from the nipple where she felt pain. She was advised to consult urgently expert doctor. When doctor had examined her and conducted few tests diagnosed her as suffering from Breast Cancer. She was given first chemotherapy followed by surgical removal of tumor and then radiation therapy. This also can be confirmed by using KP system. The star lord of ascendant Mercury is placed in third house and in quincunx with Rahu which is under aspect of Ketu; Ketu is star lord of sixth house and Rahu is star lord of twelfth house. Also, Mercury is hemmed in between Saturn and Mars which indicates occurrence of life-threatening disease and hospitalization. Further sub lord of Ascendant is Ketu placed in second house under aspect of Saturn which is sub lord of eighth cusp and occupied in thirty degrees from Mercury which is sub lord of sixth house and twelfth cusp. As such ascendant, sixth house, eighth house and twelfth house are well connected showing occurrence of cancer. When the native was required to be hospitalized in the month of November 2011 the Mahadasha of Jupiter was in progress and antardasha of Mercury was started in pratiantardasha of Ketu where Ketu is star lord of sixth house and Mercury is sub lord of sixth house. This is also noteworthy that Jupiter and Venus are under aspect of Uranus from eighth cusp which is known to cause mysterious diseases.

This was also important to note that the native was very much reluctant to visit doctor even after advising of the threat of the disease, which is commonly found in Indian women. And as such much awareness is necessary to be created amongst the females with making them understand the benefits of early diagnosis and assured recovery. In above mentioned case the native was totally recovered and even got cosmetic surgery done to eliminate the ugly look.

## Planetary Longitudes and Disposition chart

| Planets | Zodiac | Degrees | Lord of Zodiac | Star Lord | Sub Lord |
|---|---|---|---|---|---|
| Sun | Aries | 048:09:08 | Mars | Venus | Rahu |
| Moon | Taurus | 076:02:53 | Venus | Moon | Saturn |
| Mars | Gemini | 118:30:26 | Mercury | Jupiter | Venus |
| Mercury | Taurus | 067:55:06 | Venus | Sun | Venus |
| Jupiter | Aries | 045:07:02 | Mars | Venus | Venus |
| Venus | Aries | 035:30:44 | Mars | Ketu | Mars |
| Saturn | Cancer | 123:35:54 | Moon | Saturn | Saturn |
| Rahu | Libra | 229:16:31 | Venus | Rahu | Mars |
| Ketu | Aries | 049:16:31 | Mars | Venus | Rahu |
| Uranus | Libra | 221:18:14 | Venus | Rahu | Saturn |
| Neptune | Scorpio | 259:25:57 | Mars | Mercury | Venus |

## KP House Divisions and Lords of Kusp

| Cusp | Zodiac | Lord of Zodiac | Star Lord | Sub Lord |
|---|---|---|---|---|
| 01 | Pisces | Jupiter | Mercury | Ketu |
| 02 | Aries | Mars | Venus | Saturn |
| 03 | Taurus | Venus | Moon | Venus |
| 04 | Gemini | Mercury | Rahu | Venus |
| 05 | Cancer | Moon | Saturn | Moon |
| 06 | Leo | Sun | Ketu | Mercury |
| 07 | Virgo | Mercury | Moon | Mercury |
| 08 | Libra | Venus | Jupiter | Saturn |
| 09 | Scorpio | Mars | Mercury | Venus |
| 10 | Sagittarius | Jupiter | Venus | Sun |
| 11 | Capricorn | Saturn | Moon | Rahu |
| 12 | Aquarius | Saturn | Rahu | Mercury |

Case No. 056/ msd
Date of Birth 21st September 1984 at 10:32 hours in Pune with
Lat. 018:30 N Long. 073:48 E

Scorpio ascendant chart shows lord of ascendant placed in first house making
hot and strong constitution of the native. But Mars is afflicted with Ketu and
Uranus which is known to cause mysterious diseases. Also lord of fifth house

Jupiter is occupied in second house in own sign Sagittarius afflicted with Neptune and lord of third cusp and fourth cusp Saturn is placed in twelfth house conjoined with Venus which is lord of twelfth and seventh house which indicates the structural disorder related to uterus and ovaries. Also ascendant is hemmed in between Saturn and Neptune indicating abnormal growth of cells in body. Jupiter which rules growth of normal cells in body and body metabolism is afflicted with Neptune also indicates cancerous growth in body. Moon which rules the function of endocrine and exocrine glands in body and is placed in ninth house under aspect of Saturn and in quincunx with Neptune indicates structural disorders of exocrine and endocrine glands in body. Also, lord of fifth house Jupiter is under aspect of Saturn indicates malfunctioning of ovaries and hormone producing glands. Seventh house is occupied by Rahu and is under aspect of Uranus and Ketu. The breast and milk producing glands are ruled by Moon; as Moon is under aspect of Saturn gives functional disorders and Mars which rules structure of lymph nodes and lobules that produces milk is afflicted causing structural disorders of glands giving rise to growth of cancer in breast. The native visited me for seeking advice on her relationship problems with her father and brother which were strained since last few days because of some issues at their home but when the birth chart was noticed it was revealed that either native is likely to be suffering from uterine tumor or some serious health disorders which may occur in recent days. Accordingly, I discussed about health issues as the native was unmarried there was no question of immediate conception and the native told me that she is having little discomfort in breast with feeling of heaviness and hard lump felt when touched. Immediately I advised her to carry mammograph and get ensured that there is no such tumor grow. But unfortunately, when expert doctor examined her and mammograph was taken it was confirmed that small tumor of the size of about 2 centimeters was appeared in her left breast. Doctor the advised her to get operated for surgical removal of the tumor before it gets spread further. Being it was noticed in early stage the spread up was not occurred and small surgical procedure could save her from complex treatment.

According to K P system also it can be confirmed that the native had to suffer from breast cancer. Star lord of ascendant is Jupiter occupied in second cusp placed in quadrant with Sun which is star lord of sixth house, the star lord of eighth house and twelfth house is Mars occupied in first house placed in thirty degrees from Jupiter. This indicates serious structural disorders related to either uterus or breast and disorders related to ovaries functioning. The sub lord of ascendant is Rahu occupied in seventh house Mars placed in first house which is sub lord of sixth cusp also placed in quadrant with Mercury which is sub lord of eighth house with sub lord of twelfth house Sun occupied in eleventh house placed ninety degrees from Mars. Thus ascendant, sixth house, eighth cusp and twelfth cusp are well connected indicate the occurrence of the disease and hospitalization in the Dasha period of lords of sixth house. the native was hospitalized in the month of December 2013 when mahadasha of Ketu with antardasha of Mars was in progress and pratiantardasha of Ketu was just started. Planetary longitudes and disposition are given herewith.

| Planets | Zodiac | Degrees | Lord of Zodiac | Star Lord | Sub Lord |
|---|---|---|---|---|---|
| Sun | Virgo | 304:44:57 | Mercury | Sun | Saturn |
| Moon | Cancer | 250:01:24 | Moon | Saturn | Venus |
| Mars | Scorpio | 026:54:58 | Mars | Mercury | Jupiter |
| Mercury | Leo | 289:27:39 | Sun | Venus | Rahu |
| Jupiter | Sagittarius | 040:15:29 | Jupiter | Ketu | Saturn |
| Venus | Libra | 330:53:54 | Venus | Mars | Mercury |
| Saturn | Libra | 349:43:46 | Venus | Rahu | Mars |
| Rahu | Taurus | 186:54:05 | Venus | Sun | Mercury |
| Ketu | Scorpio | 006:54:05 | Mars | Saturn | Mercury |
| Uranus | Scorpio | 016:23:08 | Mars | Saturn | Jupiter |
| Neptune | Sagittarius | 035:03:01 | Jupiter | Ketu | Mars |

## KP House Divisions and Lords of cusp

| Cusp | Zodiac | Lord of Zodiac | Star Lord | Sub Lord |
|---|---|---|---|---|
| 01 | Scorpio | Mars | Jupiter | Rahu |
| 02 | Sagittarius | Jupiter | Ketu | Venus |
| 03 | Capricorn | Saturn | Sun | Jupiter |
| 04 | Aquarius | Saturn | Mars | Venus |
| 05 | Pisces | Jupiter | Saturn | Mercury |
| 06 | Aries | Mars | Ketu | Mars |
| 07 | Taurus | Venus | Sun | Jupiter |
| 08 | Gemini | Mercury | Mars | Mercury |
| 09 | Cancer | Moon | Jupiter | Rahu |
| 10 | Leo | Sun | Ketu | Moon |
| 11 | Virgo | Mercury | Sun | Mercury |
| 12 | Libra | Venus | Mars | Sun |

Case No. 057/srb
Date of birth 10th July 1976 at 15:00 hours in Raigad
Lat. 018:16 N Long. 073:46 E

Sign Libra placed in first house occupied with Uranus and Rahu and lord of ascendant occupied in tenth house afflicted with Saturn which is lord of fourth and fifth cusp indicating functional disorders of ovaries and secondary reproductive organs; Venus is also lord of eighth cusp. Sun lord of eleventh house is occupied in ninth house conjoined with Mercury which is lord of ninth and twelfth house indicates poor strength to fight with diseases and low immunity. Lord of tenth house Moon is occupied in third house with sign Sagittarius placed in quincunx with Saturn indicates functional disorders of exocrine and endocrine glands. Lord of third house Jupiter which is also lord of sixth house is placed in eighth house and under aspect of Neptune indicating growth of tumor in chest or breast. Further we can note that seventh cusp is occupied by Ketu and lord of seventh cusp Mars is placed in eleventh house in quadrant with Neptune and in triangle with Uranus cause the structural disorders of ovaries and uterus. Also, as fifth house is under aspect of Mars indicates functional disorders of uterus.

When native visited me for persistent depression syndrome along with fear of future. After observing her birth chart it was noticed that the native is passing through a phase of primary growth of some tumor in body and therefore I advised her to seek immediate medical help to confirm and treat the tumor growth so as to save her life. Doctor after examination and few tests confirmed small tumor in right side breast of about 2 centimeters across when PT scan done. First, she was treated as outpatient with chemotherapy and thereafter almost three months she was hospitalized for surgical removal of the tumor. She could save her own life only because early diagnosis and timely treatment by expert doctors.

According to K P system also it can be confirmed that just referring to the birth chart it is possible to predict the onset of life-threatening diseases and seek timely treatment. Star lord of first house is Jupiter occupied in eighth cusp which is also star lord of eighth cusp placed in quadrant with Mars which is star lord of twelfth house and in triangle with Ketu which is star lord of sixth cusp. Further sub lord of ascendant is Venus which is also sub lord of sixth cusp occupied in tenth cusp in triangle with Jupiter which is sub lord of eighth cusp and in thirty degrees from Mercury which is sub lord of twelfth cusp. this confirms the abnormal growth of cells in breast and in ovaries.

The native visited me on 18th June 2020 when mahadasha of Mars and antardasha of Venus was in progress and Ketu pratiantardasha was just started. Where Venus is sub lord of sixth house and Ketu is star lord of sixth house. Planetary Longitudes and disposition are given in below chart.

| Planet | Zodiac | Degrees | Lord of Zodiac | Star Lord | Sub Lord |
| --- | --- | --- | --- | --- | --- |
| Sun | Gemini | 264:42:37 | Mercury | Jupiter | Mercury |
| Moon | Sagittarius | 069:47:33 | Jupiter | Ketu | Saturn |
| Mars | Leo | 308:32:10 | Sun | Ketu | Jupiter |
| Mercury | Gemini | 258:28:01 | Mercury | Rahu | Moon |
| Jupiter | Taurus | 210:20:41 | Venus | Rahu | Rahu |
| Venus | Cancer | 270:49:35 | Moon | Saturn | Sun |
| Saturn | Cancer | 280:33:41 | Moon | Saturn | Sun |
| Rahu | Libra | 015:35:43 | Venus | Rahu | Venus |
| Ketu | Aries | 195:35:43 | Mars | Venus | Sun |
| Uranus | Libra | 009:30:10 | Venus | Rahu | Jupiter |
| Neptune | Scorpio | 048:08:30 | Mars | Mercury | Mercury |

## KP House Divisions and Lords of Cusp Chart

| Cusp | Zodiac | Lord of Zodiac | Star Lord | Sub Lord |
| --- | --- | --- | --- | --- |
| 01 | Libra | Venus | Jupiter | Venus |
| 02 | Scorpio | Mars | Mercury | Jupiter |
| 03 | Sagittarius | Jupiter | Sun | Sun |
| 04 | Capricorn | Saturn | Mars | Saturn |
| 05 | Pisces | Jupiter | Jupiter | Mars |
| 06 | Aries | Mars | Ketu | Venus |
| 07 | Aries | Mars | Sun | Moon |
| 08 | Taurus | Venus | Mars | Jupiter |
| 09 | Gemini | Mercury | Jupiter | Venus |
| 10 | Cancer | Moon | Mercury | Saturn |
| 11 | Virgo | Mercury | Sun | Rahu |
| 12 | Libra | Venus | Mars | Mercury |

Case No. 058/ssm
Date of Birth 02<sup>nd</sup> October 1965 at 13:10 hours. In Karimnagar
Lat. 018:24 N Long. 079:06 E

This is classic case of fight between human being with death and win over the adversaries by Human. The native came to me seek advice on persistent ill health and diseases running from behind one after the another and asked about any homam or other rituals if performed she can get relief from these diseases. The birth chart shows Sagittarius in first house with Moon occupied having Ketu as star lord od Moon and Mercury as sub lord of Moon where Mercury is also star lord of eighth cusp and twelfth cusp indicating probability of serious functional disorders associated with endocrine and exocrine glands. Lord of ascendant and fourth house is occupied in seventh cusp with sign Gemini and in quincunx with Mars and Ketu which denotes abnormal growth of cells in body leading to cancer. Saturn which is lord of second and third house is occupied in third house aspect Mars which is lord of fifth house and eighth house placed in twelfth house indicates structural disorders of uterus and ovaries. Sun which is lord of ninth house is occupied in tenth house conjoined with Mercury which is lord of seventh and tenth house indicates poor strength to fight with diseases and low immunity. Further sixth house is occupied by Rahu and lord of sixth house Venus is placed in eleventh house afflicted with Neptune, also Neptune aspect fifth house making it vulnerable for functional disorders. It also can be noticed that Uranus occupied in ninth house also denotes the growth of tumor in uterus as Uranus rules mysterious diseases. THE native when asked about any pooja or ritual to be performed for getting rid of the diseases and it was noticed that the native had already suffered from uterine adhesions and fibroids in ovaries which were operated surgically before last month. Now the native was showing further growth of tumor in left side of breast. When asked in detail it was replied that there is pain in breast with some abnormal discharge from nipples. She was therefore advised to consult expert doctor urgently as it appeared that the tumor size is consistently increasing. After examining her and conducting PT scan it was diagnosed the native was suffering from breast cancer and the tumor size had grown to approximately 4.5 centimeter across but fortunately did not spread in surrounding tissues. Doctor advised hospitalization for surgical removal of the tumor and chemotherapy. After about two months she was given radiation therapy and doctor advised her to visit initially after every six months and thereafter once in year. With reference to the reports from hospital it was learned that though lymph nodes were not affected there was tiny growth found in left side lung and poly cysts in ovaries. She was totally cured as reported on 12th January 2005 almost one year after she visited first time.

According to K P system also it can be noticed that the native was prone for disease like cancer and it is likely that this tumor may reoccur after few years probably in Rahu mahadasha November 2013 but till date the book is completed she didn't complain any thing and carry good health.

## Planetary Longitudes and Disposition chart

| Planet | Zodiac | Degrees | Lord of Zodiac | Star Lord | Sub Lord |
| --- | --- | --- | --- | --- | --- |
| Sun | Virgo | 285:31:33 | Mercury | Moon | Jupiter |
| Moon | Sagittarius | 013:15:12 | Jupiter | Ketu | Mercury |
| Mars | Scorpio | 335:14:41 | Mars | Saturn | Saturn |
| Mercury | Virgo | 289:19:39 | Mercury | Moon | Mercury |
| Jupiter | Gemini | 187:26:18 | Mercury | Rahu | Rahu |
| Venus | Libra | 328:10:00 | Venus | Jupiter | Venus |
| Saturn | Aquarius | 078:35:48 | Saturn | Rahu | Moon |
| Rahu | Taurus | 164:04:41 | Venus | Moon | Jupiter |
| Ketu | Scorpio | 344:04:41 | Mars | Saturn | Rahu |
| Uranus | Leo | 263:21:11 | Sun | Venus | Saturn |
| Neptune | Libra | 324:55:05 | Venus | Jupiter | Mercury |

## KP House Divisions and Lords of Cusp

| Cusp | Zodiac | Lord of Zodiac | Star Lord | Sub Lord |
| --- | --- | --- | --- | --- |
| 01 | Sagittarius | Jupiter | Venus | Saturn |
| 02 | Capricorn | Saturn | Mars | Rahu |
| 03 | Pisces | Jupiter | Jupiter | Mars |
| 04 | Aries | Mars | Ketu | Sun |
| 05 | Taurus | Venus | Sun | Jupiter |
| 06 | Taurus | Venus | Mars | Jupiter |
| 07 | Gemini | Mercury | Jupiter | Saturn |
| 08 | Cancer | Moon | Mercury | Rahu |
| 09 | Virgo | Mercury | Sun | Rahu |
| 10 | Libra | Venus | Mars | Venus |
| 11 | Scorpio | Mars | Jupiter | Rahu |
| 12 | Scorpio | Mars | Mercury | Jupiter |

Case No. 059/srs
Date of birth 16th December 1969 at 09:37 hours in Nagaon Assam
Lat. 027:01 N Long. 094:10 E

Capricorn sign placed in ascendant with lord of ascendant and second house placed in fourth house; lord of fourth house and eleventh house Mars is occupied in second house afflicted with Rahu indicating structural disorders of exocrine glands. Lord of seventh house Moon is placed in third house with sign Pisces and hemmed in between Mars and Saturn indicates functional disorders of endocrine and exocrine glands. Lord of eighth house Sun which rules immunity functions of body and strength to fight with diseases is occupied in twelfth house conjoined with lord of sixth house Mercury indicates uterine and ovaries disorders and diseases. Lord of third house and twelfth house Jupiter is placed in tenth house under aspect of Saturn and hemmed in between Uranus placed in ninth house and Neptune occupied in eleventh house indicates abnormal growth of cells in body. Lord of fifth house Venus is occupied in eleventh house afflicted with Neptune indicating functional disorders of ovaries and milk producing glands in breast. Also, Venus is in quincunx with Saturn and Saturn being known to cause obstructive and inflammatory disorders related to organs ruled by Venus i.e. secondary reproductive organs. Also, it can be noticed that Saturn aspect ascendant i.e. first house and causes poor immunity and strength to fight with diseases. Native came to see me after visiting TATA Cancer research center in Mumbai and was totally devastated mentally. It was then noticed the birth chart indicates hospitalization due to life threatening disease and surgical procedure is also predicted. The native was then given CBT along with short course in TA for depression disorder. According to KP system also it can be confirmed that the native is likely to suffer from tumor like disease. Star lord of ascendant is Mars placed in second house is under aspect of Jupiter which is star lord of sixth house and in triangle with Sun which is star lord of eighth and twelfth house. Further sub lord of ascendant Jupiter placed in tenth house and in quincunx with Moon which is sub lord of twelfth house and in tringle with Ketu which is sub lord of eighth house. As ascendant, sixth house, eighth house and twelfth house are well connected indicating native is prone to suffer from tumor growth followed by surgical removal and hospitalization. As the native was from high profile family and well educated did visit hospital first and then approached me. Planetary Longitudes and disposition

| Planet | Zodiac | Degrees | Lord of Zodiac | Star Lord | Sub Lord |
|---|---|---|---|---|---|
| Sun | Sagittarius | 330:35:53 | Jupiter | Ketu | Ketu |
| Moon | Pisces | 062:09:15 | Jupiter | Jupiter | Rahu |
| Mars | Aquarius | 036:59:20 | Saturn | Rahu | Rahu |
| Rahu | Sagittarius | 346:36:55 | Jupiter | Venus | Moon |
| Jupiter | Libra | 276:28:46 | Venus | Mars | Moon |
| Venus | Scorpio | 321:06:06 | Mars | Mercury | Venus |
| Saturn | Aries | 098:56:25 | Mars | Ketu | Jupiter |
| Rahu | Aquarius | 052:41:04 | Saturn | Jupiter | Saturn |
| Ketu | Leo | 232:41:04 | Sun | Venus | Saturn |
| Uranus | Virgo | 254:58:58 | Mercury | Moon | Jupiter |

## KP House Divisions and Lords of Cusp

| Cusp | Zodiac | Lord of Zodiac | Star Lord | Sub Lord |
|---|---|---|---|---|
| 01 | Capricorn | Saturn | Mars | Jupiter |
| 02 | Pisces | Jupiter | Saturn | Ketu |
| 03 | Aries | Mars | Ketu | Mercury |
| 04 | Taurus | Venus | Sun | Venus |
| 05 | Gemini | Mercury | Mars | Venus |
| 06 | Gemini | Mercury | Jupiter | Venus |
| 07 | Cancer | Moon | Mercury | Jupiter |
| 08 | Virgo | Mercury | Sun | Ketu |
| 09 | Libra | Venus | Rahu | Saturn |
| 10 | Scorpio | Mars | Saturn | Venus |
| 11 | Sagittarius | Jupiter | Ketu | Sun |
| 12 | Sagittarius | Jupiter | Sun | Moon |

Case No. 060/pas
Date of birth 23rd March 1971 at 11:00 hours in Pune
Lat. 018:30 N Long. 073:48 E

This is Taurus ascendant chart shows lord of ascendant Venus which is also lord of sixth house is placed in ninth house conjoined with Moon which is lord of third house and afflicted with Rahu also under aspect of Saturn indicates poor immunity and low strength to fight with diseases. Lord of second house and fifth house Mercury is occupied in eleventh house conjoined with Sun which is lord of fourth house and under aspect of Uranus placed in fifth house. This indicates malfunctioning of metabolism and poor immunity. Also, as lord of fifth house Mercury and lord of fourth house Sun both are under aspect of Uranus which rules mysterious diseases indicates structural disorders of ovaries and milk producing lobules in breast. Also, lord of eighth house and eleventh house Jupiter is occupied in seventh house afflicted with Neptune indicating abnormal or uncontrolled growth of cells in uterus and breasts. Lord of seventh house and twelfth house Mars is occupied in eighth house which is placed in quincunx with Ketu indicating structural disorders of uterus and breasts. Saturn which is lord of ninth house and tenth house is placed in twelfth house indicates obstructive and inflammatory diseases of tissues in body.

Native approached me in 1997 for seeking advice on severe depression and persistent pains in breast with discomfort. When I noticed the birth chart it was noticed that the native must have advanced stage of cancer and must seek immediate treatment for the same. After thorough examination doctor diagnosed her as suffering from large tumor that developed in left breast and spread into lymph nodes and accordingly advised to get hospitalized for surgical treatment followed by chemotherapy. The native got totally recovered in 1999 but again complained about pains in lower belly and pelvic region in 2018 and again got hospitalized for the treatment of uterine tumor and cancer of cervix. This can also be predicted in early stage by using K P system. Star lord of ascendant Moon is occupied in ninth house conjoined with star lord of sixth house Rahu and star lord of eighth and twelfth house Venus that confirms the occurrence of life-threatening diseases. Also sub lord of ascendant Venus is placed in ninth house conjoined with sub lord of sixth house and sub lord Moon and sub lord of twelfth house Rahu; sub lord of eighth house occupied in eighth house thirty degrees from Venus. As such ascendant, sixth house, eighth house and twelfth house are well connected indicating hospitalization, surgery and suffering. The first time disease occurred in October 1997 was in Rahu mahadasha and Moon antardasha was in progress with onset of Rahu pratiantardasha.

## Planetary longitudes and Disposition table.

| Planet | Zodiac | Degrees | Lord of Zodiac | Star Lord | Sub Lord |
|---|---|---|---|---|---|
| Sun | Pisces | 308:28:50 | Jupiter | Saturn | Venus |
| Moon | Capricorn | 258:26:13 | Saturn | Moon | Mercury |
| Mars | Sagittarius | 223:02:40 | Jupiter | Ketu | Mercury |
| Mercury | Pisces | 323:41:01 | Jupiter | Mercury | Mars |
| Jupiter | Scorpio | 192:59:55 | Mars | Saturn | Rahu |
| Venus | Capricorn | 268:59:53 | Saturn | Mars | Saturn |
| Saturn | Aries | 355:50:25 | Mars | Venus | Mercury |
| Rahu | Capricorn | 268:11:50 | Saturn | Mars | Saturn |
| Ketu | Cancer | 088:11:50 | Moon | Mercury | Saturn |
| Uranus | Virgo | 138:29:29 | Mercury | Moon | Mercury |
| Neptune | Scorpio | 189:31:50 | Mars | Saturn | Venus |

## KP House Divisions and Lords of Cusp chart

| Cusp | Zodiac | Lord of Zodiac | Star Lord | Sub Lord |
|---|---|---|---|---|
| 01 | Taurus | Venus | Moon | Venus |
| 02 | Gemini | Mercury | Rahu | Sun |
| 03 | Cancer | Moon | Saturn | Mars |
| 04 | Leo | Sun | Ketu | Saturn |
| 05 | Virgo | Mercury | Moon | Jupiter |
| 06 | Libra | Venus | Rahu | Moon |
| 07 | Scorpio | Mars | Mercury | Moon |
| 08 | Sagittarius | Jupiter | Venus | Mars |
| 09 | Capricorn | Saturn | Moon | Rahu |
| 10 | Aquarius | Saturn | Rahu | Saturn |
| 11 | Pisces | Jupiter | Saturn | Rahu |
| 12 | Aries | Mars | Venus | Rahu |

# Chapter 8

# Thyroid and Planets

Thyroid is a gland that secrets hormones which regulates energy at cellular level and play a role in many different systems throughout the body, when thyroid secretes too much or too little of these hormones it is called thyroid disorder or thyroid disease. There are several different types of thyroid diseases including hyperthyroidism, hypothyroidism and Hashimotto's thyroid.

Thyroid gland is a small organ that is in the front of neck wrapped around the windpipe or trachea. It is shaped like a butterfly, smaller portion in middle and wide wings that extends around the side of throat. The thyroid is a gland that releases hormones in the body for specific task and help control vital functions of the body. If the quantity of hormone released is more than the required it is called hyperthyroidism, and if the quantity is less it is called as hypothyroidism.

Function of thyroid, the thyroid controls metabolism with few specific hormone
1.  T4 Tetraiodothyroxine and
2.  T3 Triiodo thyroxine
3.  These two hormones are secreted by thyroid gland regulate the body cells to use energy when thyroid work properly it maintains the right amount of specific hormones to keep bods metabolism at right rate and also as the hormones used thyroid creates replacement. This is all supervised by pituitary gland located in center of the skull. Pituitary gland monitors and controls the quantity of thyroid hormones in blood stream when pituitary gland senses lack of thyroid hormone or high level of hormones in blood stream it regulates with it's own hormone called Thyroid stimulating hormone or TSH. The TSH will be sent to thyroid and thyroid will be regulated. Thyroid disease is a term for medical condition

that keeps thyroid from secreting right quantity of specific hormones. Thyroid typically secrets hormones that keep body functioning normally. When thyroid specific hormones are released in excess of specific thyroid hormone body uses energy quickly; this phenomena is called hyper thyroidism, using energy quickly make heart beat faster, cause to lose the weight without trying even make feel nervous or depressed. On the flipside of this the thyroid if secrets less too little hormone in blood stream then it is called hypothyroidism. When we have too little thyroid hormone in our body it can make us tired and might gain weight and we are unable to tolerate lower temperatures; thus two main disorders can be caused by variety of conditions and can also be genetically transferred from one generation to the next generation.

Higher risk of developing thyroid disease can be attributed to following causes.
1. Have family history of thyroid disease
2. Have medical condition like pernicious Anemia, Diabetes type 1, Lupus, Rheumatoid Arthritis, Stephan Jorgen's syndrome, Turner's syndrome Adrenal insufficiency etc.
3. Consuming medicines that contain more iodine,
4. Are older than 60 years.
5. Have had treatment for a past thyroid condition or Cancer, Thyroidectomy, Radiation.

Causes of thyroidism. Hyper thyroidism and Hypothyroidism both are caused by other diseases that impact the way the thyroid gland works.
a. The conditions that cause hypothyroidism include,
   1. Thyroiditis: it is a condition, or an inflammation of thyroid gland and thyroid gland can secrete lower quantity of thyroid in blood stream.
   2. Hashimotto's syndrome: this is a painless disease where body cell attack and damage thyroid gland and called autoimmune disease. This is genetically transmitted disease.
   3. Post-partum thyroiditis: this is temporary condition occur in about 5 to 9% of women after childbirth.
   4. Iodine deficiency syndrome: iodine is used by thyroid to generate and secrete hormones; this is most common condition found in tropical countries.

5. Nonfunctioning of thyroid gland: this is mostly congenital and often found in children, if left untreated children could have physical and mental issues in future.

b. Conditions that can cause hyperthyroidism include,

1. Greave's disease: in this disease entire thyroid gland is overactive and the problem is also called as diffuse toxic goiter or enlarged thyroid gland.

2. Nodules: hyperthyroidism is also caused by nodules that are overactive within thyroid gland; these are called nodules that secrets thyroid hormone excessively uncontrollably and work autonomously. Or a single nodule that works autonomously; with several nodules if occur called as multi toxic nodular goiter.

3. Thyroiditis: this disorder can be either painful or without pain and in this condition thyroid releases hormone that are stored some medicines like there which can last for few weeks or even months.

4. Excessive iodine: when one has too much of iodine in body thyroid makes more hormone than it needs. Excessive iodine can be found in Amiodarone used for heart ailments, and cough syrups.

Common symptoms of thyroid disorders. Experience

There are variety of symptoms one can experience if have thyroid disease. Often symptoms are remarkably like other medical conditions; and based on type are different for hyperthyroidism and Hypothyroid. For hyperthyroidism symptoms may include

1. Experiencing Anxiety, irritability, and nervousness.
2. Sleep disturbances or trouble sleeping.
3. Losing weight,
4. Having goiter or enlarged thyroid gland,
5. Having muscle weakness and tremors.
6. Experiencing irregular menstrual periods or Amenorrhea,
7. Feeling sensitive to heat,
8. Having vision problem or eye irritation.

Symptoms of hypothyroidism are as follows.

1. Fatigue,
2. Weight gain,
3. Frequent and heavy menstrual periods,

4.  Having dry hairs, or coarse hair and hair loss,
5.  Having hoarse voice,
6.  Experiencing intolerance to cold.
7.  In case of diabetes if hyperthyroidism occurs then sleepless nights and frequent urination caused.

The Thyroid disease can be predicted much earlier than it occurs if birth chart is studied so also complications due to thyroidism can also be noticed to approach doctor in time and get medications in time. With reference to the light Parashar and Kalyan Verma's Sarawali following combinations are reported so also some combinations can also be studied which were noticed during routine study of natives visited to me.

These can be summarized as given here with,
1.  Jupiter and Sun are conjoined in ascendant and are under aspect of Saturn or Uranus can cause hyperthyroidism,
2.  Uranus, Rahu, Ketu occupy first house with Sun placed in eighth house may cause hyper thyroidism.
3.  Lord of sixth house, eighth house or twelfth house occupy first house and Sun and Jupiter placed conjoined in eighth house,
4.  Sun and Saturn conjoined in fifth house with lord of ascendant occupy eighth house with Moon placed in first house with Ketu also gives hyper thyroidism,
5.  Sun conjoins Saturn in fifth house and Moon placed in seventh house with Uranus occupy first house certain to cause hyperthyroidism,
6.  Jupiter occupy twelfth cusp with Uranus conjoins Sun in first house and Saturn placed in seventh house causes hyperthyroidism,
7.  Saturn as lord of fifth house placed in eighth house conjoined with Jupiter and Mars occupy first house may cause hyperthyroidism,
8.  Ketu, Neptune occupy first house conjoined with Mars and Sun is placed in twelfth house; the native is certain to suffer from hyperthyroidism,
9.  Saturn conjoins Mars in fifth house, Rahu with Uranus are placed in first house and Jupiter occupies eighth house then native is certain to suffer from hypothyroidism or iodine deficiency syndrome.
10. Rahu conjoins Moon in first house and lord of first house is placed in eighth house causes hypothyroidism,

11. Moon placed in fifth house with lord of sixth, eighth or twelfth house and first house occupied by Saturn conjoined with Sun causes hypothyroidism,

12. Lord of eighth house placed in fifth house conjoined with Saturn or Mars and Jupiter occupies eighth house with Sun placed in sixth house certainly causes hypothyroidism,

13. Sun occupies first house with sign Aquarius and conjoins Uranus or Neptune and Saturn occupies seventh house then native is likely to suffer from hypothyroidism or thyroiditis.

14. Jupiter conjoins Saturn in first house and lord of ascendant placed in twelfth house conjoined with Mars then native is likely to suffer from Goiter or even cancer of thyroid.

15. Sun joined with Jupiter in first house, Uranus or Neptune, and Saturn occupies seventh house and Rahu placed in eighth may cause diseases related to thyroid disorders or enlargement of thyroid gland is noticed.

16. Sun placed in eighth house afflicted with Saturn and Moon occupies ascendant and under aspect of Mars and Uranus gives Goiter.

17. Jupiter and Sun conjoin in ascendant and Uranus occupies seventh house with Mars placed in tenth house with Neptune causes Thyroid diseases.

18. Sun occupies ascendant with Mars and Jupiter occupies twelfth house as lord of fifth house afflicted with Saturn or Neptune indicates thyroid diseases.

19. Lord of fifth house and Uranus occupies first house and Rahu with Mars placed in seventh house are likely to cause hypothyroidism.

20. Sun with Jupiter occupies eighth house as lord of ascendant and Mars placed in first house gives hypothyroidism.

21. Sun as lord of eighth house occupies ascendant and Jupiter placed in twelfth house with Uranus with Mars placed in second house gives hyper thyroidism.

22. In Virgo ascendant chart Sun occupies fourth house with Mars and Saturn placed in tenth house with Jupiter in sixth house with Rahu certainly gives Thyroid disorder.

23. Jupiter with Uranus occupies ascendant and lord of ascendant placed in sixth house with Uranus is likely to give Thyroid diseases.

Here we try to understand with some living examples the onset of disease and planetary disposition in birth chart.

Case No. 061/cdb
Date of Birth 14th August 1975 at 20:00 hours in Khandala
Lat. 018:03N Long. 074:01 E

This chart shows Aquarius ascendant with lord of ascendant occupied in sixth house conjoined with Sun which is lord of seventh house this indicates obstructive and inflammatory disorders in neck or brain. Jupiter which is lord of second house and eleventh house is placed in third house with sign Aries and under aspect of Uranus which is known to cause mysterious diseases and abnormal growth in body. Lord of second house and tenth house is placed in fourth house afflicted with Ketu and aspect Moon placed in tenth house which is lord of sixth house; Moon is also afflicted with Neptune and Rahu and indicates functional disorders of endocrine and exocrine glands in body also Mars indicates structural disorders of endocrine glands. Mercury which is lord of fifth house and eighth house is occupied in seventh house and conjoined with Venus which s lord of fourth and ninth house indicating functional disorders of uterus and ovaries. the native approached me in June 2016 for seeking advice on her business development and her frequent mood swing that becomes an obstacle in her business, also she complained regarding the repeated health problems she was facing recently. When her birth chart was observed it was revealed that she also must be having thyroid problems and when I asked her accordingly she replied that she had treatment for hyperthyroidism few years back and since then she had not checked again. Also, she told me that since last few months her weight had increased without any change in food habit or daily routine. I advised her to consult expert doctor from big hospital in city and then visit me. After she had doctor's consultations and clinical examination doctor diagnosed her again the same disease of hyperthyroidism. She restarted her treatment for thyroid problem and after getting cognitive behavioral therapy from me she has improved a lot and resumed her business again.

According to K P system also it can be confirmed that she had suffered from hyper Thyroidism. Star lord of first house Rahu is occupied in tenth house conjoined with Moon which is star lord of eighth house and twelfth house and Rahu aspect Saturn placed in sixth house which is star lord of sixth house. Further, Sub lord of ascendant Venus is occupied in seventh house placed in quadrant with Rahu which is sub lord of sixth house and placed in quincunx with Jupiter which is sub lord of twelfth house; Jupiter is also placed in quadrant with Sun which is sub lord of eighth house. Thus ascendant, sixth house, eighth house and twelfth house are well connected indicating thyroid malfunctioning and hospitalization for uterine and thyroid problems.

## Planetary Longitudes and Disposition chart

| Planet | Zodiac | Degrees | Lord of Zodiac | Star Lord | Sub Lord |
|---|---|---|---|---|---|
| Sun | Cancer | 177:39:59 | Moon | Mercury | Jupiter |
| Moon | Scorpio | 273:58:55 | Mars | Saturn | Saturn |
| Mars | Taurus | 096:19:04 | Venus | Sun | Mercury |
| Mercury | Leo | 190:44:43 | Sun | Ketu | Saturn |
| Jupiter | Aries | 061:11:00 | Mars | Ketu | Venus |
| Venus | Leo | 196:48:59 | Sun | Venus | Moon |
| Saturn | Cancer | 152:47:36 | Moon | Jupiter | Rahu |
| Rahu | Scorpio | 273:07:25 | Mars | Jupiter | Rahu |
| Ketu | Taurus | 093:07:25 | Venus | Sun | Saturn |
| Uranus | Libra | 245:28:22 | Venus | Mars | Sun |
| Neptune | Scorpio | 285:30:54 | Mars | Saturn | Jupiter |

## KP House Divisions and Lords of Cusp

| Planet | Zodiac | Lord of Zodiac | Star Lord | Sub Lord |
|---|---|---|---|---|
| 01 | Aquarius | Saturn | Sun | Venus |
| 02 | Pisces | Jupiter | Mercury | Moon |
| 03 | Aries | Mars | Venus | Mercury |
| 04 | Taurus | Venus | Moon | Venus |
| 05 | Gemini | Mercury | Rahu | Venus |
| 06 | Cancer | Moon | Saturn | Rahu |
| 07 | Leo | Sun | Venus | Moon |
| 08 | Virgo | Mercury | Moon | Sun |
| 09 | Libra | Venus | Jupiter | Mercury |
| 10 | Scorpio | Mars | Mercury | Sun |
| 11 | Sagittarius | Jupiter | Venus | Moon |
| 12 | Capricorn | Saturn | Moon | Jupiter |

Case No. 068/srr
Date of birth 16ᵗʰ June 1975 at 18:20 hours in Krishnagiri
Lat. 015:34 N Long. 077:49 E

Scorpio ascendant chart with Rahu conjoined with Neptune indicates malfunction of pituitary or thyroid gland. Lord of first house Mars which is also lord of sixth house is placed in fifth house conjoined with Jupiter indicates structural disorders of uterus or ovaries and abnormal growth of endocrine glands in body. Jupiter is lord of second house and fifth house and afflicted with Mars which is lord of sixth house. Sun which is lord of tenth house and which rules energy generation at cellular level in body is placed in eighth house afflicted with Saturn which is lord of third and fourth house indicates structural and functional disorders related to thyroid gland. Venus which is lord seventh house and twelfth house is placed in ninth house in quadrant with Uranus indicates ailments related to exocrine glands also. Moon which rules function of endocrine and exocrine glands in body is occupied in eleventh house and under aspect of Mars placed in fifth house, and in quadrant with Saturn placed in eighth house indicates the native is prone to suffer from endocrine and exocrine glands related diseases. Native came to me regarding sleep disturbances and was seeking solution to insomnia due to excessive thinking. But when her birth chart was observed it was noticed that there is possibility of hyperthyroidism as well as onset of diabetes and metabolism related problems. Accordingly, I advised her to consult endocrinologist and then visit me. After thorough examination and conducting essential tests doctor confirmed that the native was victim of hyperthyroidism and Diabetes associated with hypertension.

According to KP system also it can be revealed that the native is likely to be suffered from hyperthyroidism and Diabetes. As Sun which is lord of tenth cusp and star lord of sixth house it can be confirmed that metabolism is disturbed leading to problems of thyroid, diabetes and hypertension. Star lord of ascendant Mercury is occupied in seventh house placed in triangle with Jupiter which is star lord of eighth house and twelfth house. Star lord of sixth house Sun is occupied in eighth house with thirty degrees from Mercury, indicates functional disorders of endocrine secretary glands. Sub lord of ascendant is Rahu occupied in first house which is also sub lord of sixth house and aspect Mercury which is sub lord of eighth house and placed in triangle with Moon which is sub lord of eighth house. as ascendant, sixth house, eighth house and twelfth house are well connected indicate the occurrence of this disorders and need to get hospitalized. Native visited me in October 2011 when mahadasha of Rahu and antardasha of Sun was in progress and pratiantardasha of Rahu was just started.

| Planet | Zodiac | Degrees | Lord of Zodiac | Star Lord | Sub Lord |
|---|---|---|---|---|---|
| Sun | Gemini | 211:14:54 | Mercury | Mars | Mercury |
| Moon | Virgo | 300:04:03 | Mercury | Sun | Rahu |
| Mars | Pisces | 145:55:34 | Jupiter | Mercury | Rahu |
| Mercury | Taurus | 202:48:37 | Venus | Moon | Sun |
| Jupiter | Pisces | 145:57:26 | Jupiter | Mercury | Rahu |
| Venus | Cancer | 256:35:43 | Moon | Saturn | Jupiter |
| Saturn | Gemini | 235:16:47 | Mercury | Jupiter | Mercury |
| Rahu | Scorpio | 006:15:15 | Mars | Saturn | Mercury |
| Ketu | Taurus | 186:15:15 | Venus | Sun | Mercury |
| Uranus | Libra | 335:01:19 | Venus | Mars | Sun |
| Neptune | Scorpio | 016:30:22 | Mars | Saturn | Jupiter |

## KP House Divisions and Lords of Cusp

| Cusp | Zodiac | Lord of Zodiac | Star Lord | Sub Lord |
|---|---|---|---|---|
| 01 | Scorpio | Mars | Mercury | Rahu |
| 02 | Sagittarius | Jupiter | Venus | Mercury |
| 03 | Capricorn | Saturn | Mars | Rahu |
| 04 | Pisces | Jupiter | Jupiter | Rahu |
| 05 | Aries | Mars | Ketu | Sun |
| 06 | Aries | Mars | Sun | Rahu |
| 07 | Taurus | Venus | Mars | Jupiter |
| 08 | Gemini | Mercury | Jupiter | Mercury |
| 09 | Cancer | Moon | Mercury | Mercury |
| 10 | Virgo | Mercury | Sun | Mercury |
| 11 | Libra | Venus | Mars | Sun |
| 12 | Libra | Venus | Jupiter | Jupiter |

Case No. 066/ rmb
Date of birth 24ᵗʰ July 1978 at 07:30 hours in Sangola
Lat. 017:42 N Long. 075:55 E

Cancer ascendant chart is classic example of Thyroid disorder. First house is occupied by Sun which is lord of second house with sign Cancer and lord of ascendant is occupied in ninth house afflicted with Ketu indicates malfunctioning of thyroid and poor strength to fight with diseases. Moon is afflicted with Ketu and Moon rules the function of endocrine and exocrine glands and placed in quincunx with Mars and Saturn occupied in second house indicate inflammatory disease related to Thyroid gland. Jupiter which is lord of sixth and ninth house is occupied in twelfth house in quadrant with Ketu indicates abnormal growth in body and frequent hospitalization. Uranus which rules the mysterious diseases is placed in fourth house in quadrant with Sun placed in first house indicates diseases that are difficult to diagnose and weak constitution. The native approached me for frequent illness and persistent low feeling that caused drift between herself and with her husband that affected entire peace of home. She expected some thing that will eliminate the planetary ill aspect as well as Vast Doshas if at all present. When her birth chart is observed it was noticed clearly that she must have thyroid as well hormonal disorders, and I advised her to consult expert doctor to get examined. It was diagnosed by doctors that she was having enlarged thyroid gland and some fibroids developed in uterus which were causing her cranky mood and severe depression disorder. First doctor advised her to get hospitalized for removal of uterine fibroids with uterus and she was treated for enlarged thyroid with multi nodules developed into it.

According to K P system it can be conformingly predicted. Star lord of ascendant is Mercury placed in second house in thirty degrees from Sun which is star lord of sixth house and in triangle with Jupiter which is star lord of eighth house ant twelfth house. Further sub lord of ascendant Jupiter occupied in twelfth house in triangle with Mercury which is sub lord of eighth house and Venus which is sub lord of twelfth house and in thirty degrees from Sun which is sub lord of sixth house. thus ascendant, sixth house, eighth house and twelfth house are well connected indicating serious disorders of thyroid. It took almost one year to bring the disorder under control after hysterectomy; and such seriousness was effect of ignoring the primitive symptoms and misunderstandings about the mental and physical disorders.

Planetary longitudes and Disposition chart

| Planet | Zodiac | Degrees | Lord of Zodiac | Star Lord | Sub Lord |
|---|---|---|---|---|---|
| Sun | Cancer | 007:16:39 | Moon | Saturn | Mercury |
| Moon | Pisces | 241:56:57 | Jupiter | Jupiter | Rahu |
| Mars | Leo | 059:32:00 | Sun | Sun | Rahu |
| Mercury | Leo | 034:03:49 | Sun | Ketu | Moon |
| Jupiter | Gemini | 357:19:23 | Mercury | Jupiter | Venus |
| Venus | Leo | 049:58:32 | Sun | Venus | Rahu |
| Saturn | Leo | 036:09:28 | Sun | Ketu | Rahu |
| Rahu | Virgo | 066:11:20 | Mercury | Sun | Mercury |
| Ketu | Pisces | 3246:11:20 | Jupiter | Saturn | Mercury |
| Uranus | Libra | 108:45:42 | Venus | Rahu | Moon |
| Neptune | Scorpio | 142:18:07 | Mars | Mercury | Moon |

Case No. 069/spg
Date of birth 11ᵗʰ August 1973 at 20:01 hours in Pune
Lat. 018:30 N Long. 073:38 E

This native being highly qualified and civilized was expected to pay an attention to self-health but unfortunately it did not happen. Native came to me in January 2003 for some psychological issues and solutions to those issues, but when her birth chart was studied it was clearly noticed that she must be having some issues with Thyroid or is likely to face in recent future. In chart with Aquarius ascendant lord of ascendant Saturn which is also lord of twelfth house is placed in fifth house afflicted with Ketu indicates diseases related to reproductive system and obstructive and inflammatory disorders of uterus. Sun, which is lord of seventh house and which rules metabolism in body and imparts immunity and strength to fight with diseases is placed in sixth house conjoined with Mercury which is lord of eighth house and lord of fifth house indicates disturbed metabolism and poor strength to fight with diseases. Jupiter which rules the growth of body cells and lord of second and eleventh house is occupied in twelfth house in quincunx with Saturn and Ketu and also in quadrant with Mars in third house indicates abnormal cell growth in body and also causes functional disorders of thyroid gland. Moon lord of sixth house and that rules function of endocrine glands and exocrine glands in body is placed afflicted with Rahu in eleventh house under aspect of Saturn and

Ketu indicates functional disorders of endocrine and exocrine glands in body. Further Venus which rules uterus and secondary reproductive organs in body is placed in seventh house in quadrant with Neptune and under aspect of Saturn indicates structural and functional disorders of uterus and ovaries. When native was advised to seek doctors and experts immediately, she was initially stunned saying she does not have any health issues except sleep disorder and excessive weight gain but agreed to consult doctor for routine examination. Doctor when examined her firstly her blood pressure was as high as 160/90 as against normal of 120/80 and therefore conducted certain tests which revealed that she was having hyper thyroidism and other issues related to liver function and obesity. She was treated as outpatient for almost four months and then doctor admitted her to hospital for removal of uterus accordingly, she got totally recovered after almost six months i.e. in August 2003.

## Planetary Longitudes and Disposition

| Planet | Zodiac | Degrees | Lord of Zodiac | Star Lord | Sub Lord |
| --- | --- | --- | --- | --- | --- |
| Sun | Cancer | 175:16:27 | Moon | Mercury | Rahu |
| Moon | Sagittarius | 327:18:31 | Jupiter | Sun | Sun |
| Mars | Aries | 066:03:38 | Mars | Ketu | Rahu |
| Mercury | Cancer | 156:37:07 | Moon | Saturn | Mercury |
| Jupiter | Capricorn | 342:10:12 | Saturn | Moon | Rahu |
| Venus | Leo | 207:35:58 | Sun | Sun | Moon |
| Saturn | Gemini | 127:32:06 | Mercury | Rahu | Rahu |
| Rahu | Sagittarius | 311:57:58 | Jupiter | Ketu | Mercury |
| Ketu | Gemini | 131:57:58 | Mercury | Rahu | Saturn |
| Uranus | Virgo | 236:20:09 | Mercury | Mars | Jupiter |
| Neptune | Scorpio | 281:10:49 | Mars | Saturn | Moon |

## KP House Divisions and Lords of Cusp

| Cusp | Zodiac | Lord of Zodiac | Star Lord | Sub Lord |
| --- | --- | --- | --- | --- |
| 01 | Aquarius | Saturn | Rahu | Mercury |
| 02 | Pisces | Jupiter | Mercury | Venus |
| 03 | Aries | Mars | Venus | Saturn |
| 04 | Taurus | Venus | Moon | Mercury |
| 05 | Gemini | Mercury | Rahu | Ketu |
| 06 | Cancer | Moon | Saturn | Moon |

| Cusp | Zodiac | Lord of Zodiac | Star Lord | Sub Lord |
| --- | --- | --- | --- | --- |
| 07 | Leo | Sun | Venus | Venus |
| 08 | Virgo | Mercury | Moon | Venus |
| 09 | Libra | Venus | Jupiter | Saturn |
| 10 | Scorpio | Mars | Mercury | Venus |
| 11 | Sagittarius | Jupiter | Venus | Venus |
| 12 | Capricorn | Saturn | Moon | Mars |

Case No. 070/shj
Date of birth 09<sup>th</sup> February 1973 at 08:11 hours in Barshi
Lat. 018:12 N Long. 075:42 E

Aquarius ascendant chart with lord of ascendant and Twelfth house Saturn placed in fourth house under aspect of Neptune occupied in tenth house indicates obstructive and inflammatory disorders. Mercury which is lord of eighth house and fifth house is occupied in first house under aspect of Saturn and in quadrant with Neptune indicates structural disorders of epithelial lining of reproductive system. Moon lord of sixth house which rules endocrine and exocrine glands is occupied in third house in quincunx with Neptune and under aspect of Rahu. This indicates disorders related to thyroid, ovaries and pituitary glands. Sun which rules strength to fight with diseases and immunity in body is placed in twelfth cusp conjoined with Jupiter which is lord of eleventh house and second house and with Venus which is lord of fourth and ninth house. Sun is placed in triangle with Neptune and in quincunx with Ketu indicates poor immunity and metabolic disorders. Jupiter which rules growth of cells is also placed in twelfth house and in quincunx with Ketu indicates abnormal growth of cells in body. Venus rules secondary reproductive system and is placed in twelfth house in quincunx with Ketu indicates structural and functional disorders of uterus and ovaries. Also, Venus placed in Capricorn in twelfth house denotes functional disorders of pancreas. As first house is in quincunx with Uranus placed in eighth house causes thyroid disorders. The native visited me in November 2007 for repeated health problems and sleep disorder. When birth chart was studied it was observed that native must have chronic disorder related to uterus and hyperthyroidism. Accordingly, when discussed in detail she told me that she was suffering from persistent weight gain and consuming regularly tablets for hypertension and insomnia. Also, the menstrual periods were irregular and with severe pain in back. I advised her to visit hospital and consult endocrinologist for thyroid or even prediabetic stage. Doctor after examining her and conducting few tests confirmed she was having hyper thyroidism and metabolic disorders, she was also asked to talk to gynecologist and get examined. Gynecologist also confirmed the adhesions in uterus and chronic pelvic inflammation disease. After almost four months native came to me and was very fresh looking and happy. Basically, she was required to continue medicines for hyperthyroidism, but other problems were over; even menstruation disorders also were recovered. This happens only because normally female diseases are taken lightly and ignored totally. When any disease becomes chronic it becomes difficult to treat and even to diagnose as initially doctors advised her only medicines for hypertension but root cause of hypertension was not traced and when doctor diagnosed exact cause of the hypertension there was no hypertension. It is evident by looking these few cases that in any society the female health is almost ignored by other family members and native herself ignores or out of fear avoid visiting doctors. In this case also KP system can even be used to predict the onset of disease and nature of the disease. Star lord of ascendant is Rahu occupied in eleventh house placed in quincunx with Saturn which is star lord of sixth house and conjoined with Mars which is star lord of eighth house. star lord of twelfth house Moon is occupied in third house with sign Aries owned by Mars. Further Sub lord of first house is Sun occupied in twelfth house conjoined with Jupiter which is sub lord of sixth house and twelfth house and placed in thirty degrees from Rahu indicates the thyroid related diseases and chronic disorders.

## Planetary Longitudes and Disposition

| Planet | Zodiac | Degrees | Lord of Zodiac | Star Lord | Sub Lord |
| --- | --- | --- | --- | --- | --- |
| Sun | Capricorn | 356:43:59 | Saturn | Mars | Jupiter |
| Moon | Aries | 067:33:11 | Mars | Ketu | Rahu |
| Mars | Sagittarius | 304:20:00 | Jupiter | Ketu | Moon |
| Mercury | Aquarius | 005:19:51 | Saturn | Mars | Sun |
| Jupiter | Capricorn | 333:23:04 | Saturn | Sun | Saturn |
| Venus | Capricorn | 341:56:02 | Venus | Moon | Rahu |
| Saturn | Taurus | 110:10:02 | Venus | Moon | Ketu |
| Rahu | Sagittarius | 321:41:23 | Jupiter | Venus | Jupiter |
| Ketu | Gemini | 141:41:23 | Mercury | Jupiter | Jupiter |
| Uranus | Virgo | 239:29:57 | Mercury | Mars | Saturn |
| Neptune | Scorpio | 283:43:25 | Mars | Saturn | Rahu |

KP House Divisions and Lords of Cusp

| Cusp | Zodiac | Lord of Zodiac | Star Lord | Sub Lord |
| --- | --- | --- | --- | --- |
| 01 | Aquarius | Saturn | Rahu | Sun |
| 02 | Pisces | Jupiter | Mercury | Rahu |
| 03 | Aries | Mars | Venus | Ketu |
| 04 | Taurus | Venus | Moon | Sun |
| 05 | Gemini | Mercury | Rahu | Sun |
| 06 | Cancer | Moon | Saturn | Jupiter |
| 07 | Leo | Sun | Venus | Mars |
| 08 | Virgo | Mercury | Mars | Rahu |
| 09 | Libra | Venus | Jupiter | Ketu |
| 10 | Scorpio | Mars | Mercury | Moon |
| 11 | Sagittarius | Jupiter | Venus | Mars |
| 12 | Capricorn | Saturn | Moon | Jupiter |

Case No. 062/gur

Date of Birth 26th June 1966 at 05:55 hours in Mumbai

Lat. 019:02 N Long. 072:50 E

This is Gemini ascendant chart with lord of ascendant falls in second house with Cancer sign and first house is occupied by Sun which is lord of third house placed in quadrant with Saturn placed in fourth house and in quincunx with Ketu occupied in fifth house indicates poor immunity and strength to fight with diseases; Sun is conjoined with Jupiter which is lord of tenth house and third house which rules growth of cells is also in quadrant with Saturn and quincunx with Ketu causes abnormal growth of thyroid gland. Moon which rules function of endocrine and exocrine glands is placed in fourth house under aspect of Saturn and in quincunx with Rahu occupied in eleventh house indicates functional disorders of endocrine and exocrine glands. Saturn which is lord of eighth house occupied in tenth house is in quincunx with fifth house gives disorders related with uterus and ovaries. Also, lord of sixth house Mars is placed in twelfth house conjoined with Venus which is lord of fifth house indicates structural and functional disorders of uterus and ovaries. The native visited me for seeking some solution on her personal relationship problems with her husband and was very much tired and depressed also because of post-menopausal syndrome, she was already detected hypertension and was under treatment for hypertension. When her birth chart was noticed first thing observed was weak constitution and exceptionally low mental strength to fight with diseases. Also, it was noticed that Sun and Jupiter in quadrant with Saturn were indicating post-menopausal thyroid hyperactivity. After discussion with her she disclosed everything she wanted to share with me and asked for help. First thing that was required to have expert opinion on the thyroid functioning. Accordingly, I advised her to consult gynecologist and seek advice on post-menopausal possibility of thyroid malfunctioning and if required consultation with endocrinologist. After conducting different tests and examinations doctor confirmed onset of hyperthyroidism due to Lupus and Rheumatoid Arthritis which was already present.

Then doctor advised certain course of long-term treatment. According to K P system also it can be predicted. Star lord of first house Rahu is occupied in eleventh house in triangle with Sun which is star lord of eighth and twelfth house and Saturn occupied in tenth house in quadrant with Sun. Also sub lord of ascendant Rahu is occupied in eleventh house placed in quadrant with Mercury which is sub lord of sixth house and twelfth house and Jupiter which is sub lord of eighth house placed in Gemini owned by Mercury. Thus ascendant, sixth house, eighth house and twelfth house are well connected indicating the thyroid and Rheumatoid arthritis. The native visited me in the month of February 2013 and according to her she must have started suffering symptoms of Thyroid before that month, when mahadasha of Saturn and antardasha of Mercury was in progress and pratiantardasha of Saturn was started.

Planetary Longitudes and Disposition chart

| Planet | Zodiac | Degrees | Lord of Zodiac | Star Lord | Sub Lord |
|---|---|---|---|---|---|
| Sun | Gemini | 010:35:06 | Mercury | Rahu | Saturn |
| Moon | Virgo | 106:36:32 | Mercury | Moon | Saturn |
| Mars | Taurus | 356:17:55 | Venus | Mars | Jupiter |
| Mercury | Cancer | 035:41:55 | Moon | Saturn | Mercury |
| Jupiter | Gemini | 017:32:44 | Mercury | Rahu | Sun |
| Venus | Taurus | 336:03:49 | Venus | Sun | Mercury |
| Saturn | Pisces | 276:06:11 | Jupiter | Saturn | Mercury |
| Rahu | Aries | 329:56:40 | Mars | Sun | Rahu |
| Ketu | Libra | 149:56:40 | Venus | Jupiter | Moon |
| Uranus | Leo | 082:35:03 | Sun | Venus | Saturn |
| Neptune | Libra | 146:21:08 | Venus | Jupiter | Ketu |

This is interesting here to note that Star lord of Sun is Rahu is also star lord of Jupiter indicating certainty of occurrence of thyroid.

KP House Divisions and Lords of Cusp

| Cusp | Zodiac | Lord of Zodiac | Star Lord | Sub Lord |
|---|---|---|---|---|
| 01 | Gemini | Mercury | Rahu | Rahu |
| 02 | Cancer | Moon | Jupiter | Rahu |
| 03 | Cancer | Moon | Mercury | Saturn |
| 04 | Leo | Sun | Sun | Mars |
| 05 | Libra | Venus | Mars | Ketu |
| 06 | Scorpio | Mars | Saturn | Mercury |
| 07 | Sagittarius | Jupiter | Ketu | Jupiter |
| 08 | Capricorn | Saturn | Sun | Jupiter |
| 09 | Capricorn | Saturn | Mars | Saturn |
| 10 | Aquarius | Saturn | Jupiter | Sun |
| 11 | Aries | Mars | Ketu | Venus |
| 12 | Taurus | Venus | Sun | Mercury |

Case No. 071/svr
Date of birth 13th April 1978 at 02:00 hours in Pune
Lat. 018:30 N Long. 073:48 E

This is classic case of hyperthyroidism and with late diagnosis only due to fear factor which prevented the native to visit Doctor. With sign Capricorn placed in ascendant and lord of ascendant and second house occupied in eighth house indicates weak constitution and somewhat depressed personality. Sun which rules the vigor and vitality in body and imparts strength to fight with diseases is occupied in third house with sign Pisces afflicted with Ketu also gives poor immunity and poor strength to fight with diseases. Also lord of sixth house Mercury is conjoined with Sun in third house indicating health problems related to pituitary gland and nervous system. Sun is also lord of eighth house and placed in quincunx with Saturn. Venus which rules function of secondary reproductive system is occupied fourth house in quadrant with Mars and under aspect of Uranus which is known to cause mysterious diseases, indicates functional disorders of ovaries and uterus. Mars which is lord of fourth and eleventh house is placed in seventh house and in quadrant with Uranus indicates structural disorders of uterus and ovaries. Lord of seventh house Moon is occupied in fifth house under aspect of Saturn and Neptune placed in eleventh house; as Moon rules the endocrine and exocrine glands and as is debilitated indicates functional disorders of endocrine and exocrine glands. Also, Moon is placed in quincunx with Uranus indicates thyroid malfunctioning and ovaries malfunctioning. Sun placed in third house is also in quincunx with Saturn and under aspect of Rahu clearly indicates hyperthyroidism. The native came to me in 2016 for problem related to her cranky and swinging mood disorder and her continued quarrels with her husband. When her birth chart was observed it was noticed that she must be experiencing anxiety, irritability and nervousness and hyper thyroidism and problems related to her menstruation cycle. Also, it was noticed that she was suffering from severe hair loss and as such I advised her to get expert medical help for probable thyroid disorder and hormonal disorder. Doctors after examining her and conducting few tests confirmed hyperthyroidism associated with hormonal disorders. She was required to get hospitalized for about weeks' time and after almost she visited to me for expressing thanks. She appeared to be changed totally with fresh look. According to K P system also it can be predicted the hyperthyroidism and uterus related disease. Star lord of first house is Sun placed in third cusp under aspect of Rahu which is star lord of sixth cusp and conjoined with Ketu which is star lord of twelfth cusp, Venus which is star lord of eighth cusp is placed in thirty degrees from Sun and Rahu. Further sub lord of ascendant and sub lord of eighth house Venus is placed in fourth house Saturn, sub lord of sixth house placed in eighth house in quincunx with Mercury which is sub lord of twelfth house. Mercury is placed in third house in thirty degrees with Venus. This indicates malfunctioning of thyroid and ovaries requiring hospitalization. Thus native had to suffer from thyroid disorders but could have been avoided if she had taken care at an early stage.

Planetary longitudes and disposition chart is tabled on next page.

## Planetary Longitudes and Disposition

| Planet | Zodiac | Degrees | Lord of Zodiac | Star Lord | Sub Lord |
|---|---|---|---|---|---|
| Sun | Pisces | 089:00:54 | Jupiter | Mercury | Saturn |
| Moon | Taurus | 149:13:55 | Venus | Mars | Saturn |
| Mars | Cancer | 187:10:33 | Moon | Saturn | Mercury |
| Mercury | Pisces | 087:00:41 | Jupiter | Mercury | Jupiter |
| Jupiter | Gemini | 156:33:57 | Mercury | Mars | Moon |
| Venus | Aries | 108:43:30 | Mars | Venus | Rahu |
| Saturn | Leo | 210:14:20 | Sun | Ketu | Ketu |
| Rahu | Virgo | 251:36:22 | Mercury | Moon | Mars |
| Ketu | Pisces | 071:36:22 | Jupiter | Saturn | Moon |
| Uranus | Libra | 291:44:57 | Venus | Jupiter | Jupiter |
| Neptune | Scorpio | 324:37:29 | Mars | Mercury | Saturn |

## KP House Divisions and Lords of cusp

| Cusp | Zodiac | Lord of Zodiac | Star Lord | Sub Lord |
|---|---|---|---|---|
| 01 | Capricorn | Saturn | Sun | Venus |
| 02 | Aquarius | Saturn | Rahu | Ketu |
| 03 | Pisces | Jupiter | Mercury | Venus |
| 04 | Aries | Mars | Venus | Jupiter |
| 05 | Taurus | Venus | Moon | Saturn |
| 06 | Gemini | Mercury | Rahu | Saturn |
| 07 | Cancer | Moon | Saturn | Venus |
| 08 | Leo | Sun | Venus | Venus |
| 09 | Virgo | Mercury | Moon | Ketu |
| 10 | Libra | Venus | Jupiter | Jupiter |
| 11 | Scorpio | Mars | Mercury | Mercury |
| 12 | Sagittarius | Jupiter | Ketu | Mercury |

Case No. 064/ksr

Date of birth 09th January 1982 at 06:40 hours. In Mumbai at Lat. 018:57 N Long. 072:49 E

Sagittarius placed in first house occupying Sun which is lord of eighth house afflicted with Ketu and Neptune. Sun rules immunity, vigor and vitality and is afflicted with Neptune indicating poor strength to fight with diseases and poor immunity. Lord of ascendant, Jupiter is occupied in eleventh house hemmed in between Uranus and Saturn, indicates abnormal growth of cells in body also causes underactive thyroid. Moon which rules endocrine and exocrine glands in body is occupied in seventh house afflicted with Rahu and under aspect of Ketu and Neptune, this indicate functional disorders of endocrine and exocrine glands. Lord of fifth house Mars is placed in tenth house afflicted with Saturn and in quadrant with Rahu and Keu indicates functional disorders of uterus and ovaries.

The native came to me for persistent low feeling and excessive sleep, she was constantly experiencing intolerance to cold, and complained regarding dry and coarse hair with short menses and heavy menstrual periods. She was asked to consult doctor for early diagnosis and treatment. Doctor after examination and conducting few tests confirmed she was suffering from hypothyroidism and iodine deficiency syndrome. Her treatment was continued for almost 2 years and recently she visited me last month for sharing her experiences and appeared to be very fresh and much better than previous. According to KP system also it can be noticed that the native is likely to be suffered form thyroid disorders. Star Lord of first house Venus is occupied in second house conjoined with star lord of eighth house and twelfth house and star lord of sixth house Moon is placed in quincunx with Venus. Also, sub lord of ascendant is Sun placed in first house and in thirty degrees from Venus and Mercury, as such first hose, sixth house, eighth house and twelfth house are well connected indicate thyroid disorders.

Planetary Longitudes and Disposition chart

| Planet | Zodiac | Degrees | Lord of Zodiac | Star Lord | Sub Lord |
|---|---|---|---|---|---|
| Sun | Sagittarius | 024:50:32 | Jupiter | Venus | Mercury |
| Moon | Gemini | 193:59:33 | Mercury | Rahu | Mercury |
| Mars | Virgo | 286:35:23 | Mercury | Moon | Saturn |
| Mercury | Capricorn | 041:32:03 | Saturn | Moon | Mars |
| Jupiter | Libra | 313:34:30 | Venus | Rahu | Mercury |
| Venus | Capricorn | 043:53:33 | Saturn | Moon | Jupiter |
| Saturn | Virgo | 298:12:36 | Mercury | Mars | Saturn |
| Rahu | Gemini | 209:09:37 | Mercury | Jupiter | Sun |
| Ketu | Sagittarius | 029:09:37 | Jupiter | Sun | Mars |
| Uranus | Scorpio | 339:29:33 | Mars | Saturn | Venus |
| Neptune | Sagittarius | 001:50:15 | Jupiter | Ketu | Venus |

## KP House Divisions and Lords of Cusp

| Cusp | Zodiac | Lord of Zodiac | Star Lord | Sub Lord |
|---|---|---|---|---|
| 01 | Sagittarius | Jupiter | Venus | Sun |
| 02 | Capricorn | Saturn | Moon | Mercury |
| 03 | Aquarius | Saturn | Jupiter | Saturn |
| 04 | Pisces | Jupiter | Mercury | Jupiter |
| 05 | Aries | Mars | Venus | Mercury |
| 06 | Taurus | Venus | Moon | Venus |
| 07 | Gemini | Mercury | Rahu | Venus |
| 08 | Cancer | Moon | Mercury | Mercury |
| 09 | Leo | Sun | Venus | Saturn |
| 10 | Virgo | Mercury | Mars | Jupiter |
| 11 | Libra | Venus | Jupiter | Mercury |
| 12 | Scorpio | Mars | Mercury | Venus |

Case No. 072/ssl
Date of birth 28th December 1988 at 09:50 hours in Buldhana
Lat. 020:21 N Long. 076:15 E

Capricorn placed in first house with lord of ascendant occupied in twelfth house conjoined with Sun which is lord of eighth house and Mercury which is lord of sixth and ninth house and afflicted with Uranus and Neptune. Sun rules the strength to fight with diseases and metabolism in body is afflicted with Uranus and Neptune indicating poor immunity and weak constitution. Mercury which rules epithelial lining of the internal organs and nervous system occupied with Sun indicates disorders related to nervous system and lining of uterus. Lord of first house occupied in twelfth house afflicted with Uranus and Neptune indicates obstructive and inflammatory diseases. Lord of twelfth house and third house Jupiter is occupied in fifth house placed in quincunx with Uranus and Neptune indicates abnormal growth of cells in body and inflammation of Lymph nodes in body. Moon which rules function of endocrine and exocrine glands in body and lord of seventh house is occupied in eighth house afflicted with Ketu indicates serious problems related with endocrine and exocrine glands. Mars which rules body fluids and blood in body is occupied in third house placed in quadrant with Uranus and Neptune indicates malfunctioning of fluid producing gland and blood disorders in body.

The native approached me in February 2016 for seeking some solution to her financial problems and regarding her recently disturbed mental condition. When her birth chart is observed it was noticed that she must be having some problems related to her health especially thyroid and menstruation cycle and when asked about she replied that since last few months she is carrying some or the other problems related to her health, complained of anxiety, sleepless nights, and muscle weakness. She also complained regarding absence of menstrual periods since last three months. When her birth chart was observed it was cleared that she must be having problems related to thyroid and other endocrine glands and therefore was advised to consult doctor immediately. When doctor examined her and conducted few tests, diagnosed enlargement of thyroid and fibroids in ovaries. According to K P System also it can be predicted that the native is suffering from thyroid and other endocrine glands. The native visited me in the month of February 2016 and was confirmed of having thyroid disorder in the month of March 2016 when Sun mahadasha and Venus antardasha was in progress and Jupiter pratiantardasha was about to finish.

Planetary Longitudes and Disposition chart

| Planet | Zodiac | Degrees | Lord of Zodiac | Star Lord | Sub lord |
| --- | --- | --- | --- | --- | --- |
| Sun | Sagittarius | 342:57:06 | Jupiter | Ketu | Mercury |
| Moon | Leo | 220:13:46 | Sun | Ketu | Saturn |
| Mars | Pisces | 084:34:38 | Jupiter | Mercury | Rahu |
| 4Mercury | Sagittarius | 355:50:51 | Jupiter | Sun | Moon |
| Jupiter | Taurus | 123:17:26 | Venus | Sun | Saturn |
| Venus | Scorpio | 319:19:00 | Mars | Mercury | Ketu |
| Saturn | Sagittarius | 341:26:15 | Jupiter | Ketu | Saturn |
| Rahu | Aquarius | 044:16:56 | Saturn | Rahu | Mercury |
| Ketu | Leo | 224:16:56 | Sun | Venus | Venus |
| Uranus | Sagittarius | 337:49:10 | Jupiter | Ketu | Jupiter |
| Neptune | Sagittarius | 346:04:21 | Jupiter | Venus | Sun |

KP House Divisions and Lords of Cusp chart is tabled on next page.

KP House Divisions and Lords of Cusp Chart

| Cusp | Zodiac | Lord of Zodiac | Star Lord | Sub Lord |
| --- | --- | --- | --- | --- |
| 01 | Capricorn | Saturn | Mars | Jupiter |
| 02 | Pisces | Jupiter | Saturn | Saturn |
| 03 | Aries | Mars | Ketu | Jupiter |
| 04 | Taurus | Venus | Sun | Mercury |
| 05 | Gemini | Mercury | Mars | Mercury |
| 06 | Gemini | Mercury | Jupiter | Venus |
| 07 | Cancer | Moon | Mercury | Jupiter |
| 08 | Virgo | Mercury | Sun | Saturn |
| 09 | Libra | Venus | Rahu | Rahu |
| 10 | Scorpio | Mars | Saturn | Mercury |
| 11 | Sagittarius | Jupiter | Ketu | Venus |
| 12 | Sagittarius | Jupiter | Sun | Sun |

Case No. 061/ cdb
Date of Birth 15<sup>th</sup> August 1978 at 22:00 hours in Mumbai
Lat. 018:57 N Long. 072:49 E

Sign Leo placed in ascendant with lord of ascendant occupied in sixth house conjoined with Venus which is lord of third and tenth cusp and lord of sixth house Saturn occupied in ascendant which indicate poor immunity and low strength to fight with diseases. Also first house and Saturn are hemmed in between Mars and Rahu indicate obstructive and inflammatory diseases. Moon which rules function of endocrine and exocrine glands is occupied in eighth house afflicted with Ketu indicates disorders of endocrine and exocrine glands in body. Further Jupiter which rules growth of cells in body is occupied in eleventh house; Jupiter is lord of eighth and fifth house placed in quadrant with Rahu and Ketu indicates abnormal growth of cells in body. Mercury which rules epithelial lining of uterus and nervous system is placed in fifth house and is in quincunx with Mars and in quadrant with Rahu and Ketu indicate inflammatory diseases and infection of lining of uterus. As lord of sixth house Saturn occupied in first house and further it is hemmed in between Mars and Rahu causes chronic diseases and obstructive disorders of ovaries and thyroid gland.

When native visited me in August 2016 was suffering from irritability, frequent mood swing and frequent quarrels with her husband on exceedingly small issues. Fortunately, her husband had also accompanied her. When her birth chart was understood, it was noticed that she must be having thyroid related disorders and also must be having some issues related to menstruation periods, when asked she replied that minor issues are there but major issues are only psychological. I advised her to consult expert endocrinologist or gynecologist, and then come to me for advice. Accordingly, she went to her gynecologist and got herself tested, Doctor after examination and conducting few tests confirmed Hypothyroidism and adhesions in uterus. She was initially treated as outpatient and afterwards admitted to hospital for hysterectomy. After almost four months she again visited me for expressing thanks, when she was fresh and healthy looking. In this case was completely unaware of thyroid problem and was assuming it was her mentality changed. According to K P System also it can be confirmed she was having thyroid related problem. Star lord of first house Venus is placed in sixth house, in thirty degrees with Mercury which is star lord of eighth and twelfth house and in triangle with Moon which is star lord of sixth house. Sub lord of ascendant Saturn is occupied in first house in quincunx with Sun which is sub lord of sixth house and Venus which is sub lord of eighth house. Also Moon which is sub lord of twelfth house is occupied in eighth house in quincunx with Saturn. As such ascendant, sixth cusp, eighth cusp and twelfth house are well connected indicating disorders of thyroid. Moon is star lord of sixth house and Sun is sub lord of sixth house.

in this classic example Moon, Sun and Jupiter all are either afflicted or under aspect of malefic planets and this caused difficulty in diagnosis and also due to unawareness in native family about the female problems she was treated as if she deliberately quarrels with her husband, mother in law and father in law, creating unnecessary complications in relation and spoiling the peace of house. and this disorder could have exponentially grown to create threat to life of native. It is therefore necessary to make every female understand the change in their behavior may have link with their personal health and required to seek immediate help of expert doctors for the same.

## Planetary Longitudes and Disposition chart

| Planet | Zodiac | Degrees | Lord of Zodiac | Star Lord | Sub Lord |
|---|---|---|---|---|---|
| Sun | Capricorn | 151:37:52 | Saturn | Sun | Jupiter |
| Moon | Pisces | 238:34:30 | Jupiter | Mercury | Jupiter |
| Mars | Cancer | 340:34:33 | Moon | Saturn | Sun |
| Mercury | Sagittarius | 128:35:09 | Jupiter | Ketu | Jupiter |
| Jupiter | Gemini | 304:32:02 | Mercury | Mars | Venus |
| Venus | Capricorn | 150:03:32 | Saturn | Sun | Rahu |
| Saturn | Leo | 005:53:46 | Sun | Ketu | Rahu |
| Rahu | Virgo | 046:13:28 | Mercury | Moon | Saturn |
| Ketu | Pisces | 226:13:28 | Jupiter | Saturn | Jupiter |
| Uranus | Libra | 082:18:04 | Venus | Jupiter | Saturn |
| Neptune | Scorpio | 113:41:00 | Mars | Mercury | Mars |

## KP House Divisions and Lords of Cusp

| Cusp | Zodiac | Lord of Zodiac | Star Lord | Sub Lord |
|---|---|---|---|---|
| 01 | Leo | Sun | Venus | Saturn |
| 02 | Virgo | Mercury | Moon | Venus |
| 03 | Libra | Venus | Jupiter | Saturn |
| 04 | Scorpio | Mars | Mercury | Moon |
| 05 | Sagittarius | Jupiter | Venus | Saturn |
| 06 | Capricorn | Saturn | Moon | Sun |
| 07 | Aquarius | Saturn | Jupiter | Saturn |
| 08 | Pisces | Jupiter | Mercury | Venus |
| 09 | Aries | Mars | Venus | Saturn |
| 10 | Taurus | Venus | Moon | Sun |
| 11 | Gemini | Mercury | Jupiter | Saturn |
| 12 | Cancer | Moon | Mercury | Moon |

# Chapter 9

# What Must We Learn?

It is need of this hour that everybody of us should try to create an awareness amongst our sisters, mother, daughters, or other relatives regarding their health issues to take advantage of latest developments of modern medical science. Each year, the American Cancer Society estimates the numbers of New Cancer cases and deaths that will occur in United States and complies the most recent data on population-based Cancer occurrence. Incidence data through 2016 were collected by surveillance, Epidemiology and End result program, the National Program of Cancer Registries and the North American

Association of Central Cancer Registries; mortality data were through 2017 were collected. National Centre for Health Statistics in 2018 were having total 1,806,590 new Cancer cases and 606,520 deaths were projected to occur. When actual data of deaths due to Cancer was studied it was clearly noticed that 74% deaths were due to uterine and breast Cancer only and surprisingly it was also revealed that of these 40% deaths could have been avoided by creating an awareness in women to notice the early signs of occurrence of Cancer. in India though the exact data is not available, but it can be believed that the situation in India is still worse as our society is based on various beliefs and faith with different values of life which makes an Indian woman to ignore the health signs that may help us save their lives. This was observed by one large Hospital in Capital of Delhi and the data collected was an eye opener describing almost 70% of the women cancer cases are result of delayed diagnosis and lack of awareness in females regarding this life-threatening disease. When I was in one remote south city cum village Suchindram In Kerala it was interesting to chat with the life style of those people and during our chat many people told me that many females in the village are having the major PID (Pelvic Inflammation Disease) issues and now most of these females are habitat to the pains and other symptoms, which was shocking and was revealed by a Doctor from the village as he is having his good practice in the village. Like this wherever I have had chat with health care professionals from various villages in India same thing was noticed; surprisingly even after doctor advises the patients to get examined and conduct few test they avoided it not because financial issues but because of shear fear factor.

Health Care professionals in India have this biggest challenge before them and we all shall have to take it seriously to create awareness about female health.

I hope this book will help my health Care friends to promote awareness in female health issues so that our coming generation will certainly be healthy and free from life time sufferings like Autism, Cerebral Palsy and many more.

9 781649 838308